Operational research in tropical and other communicable diseases

Final Report Summaries 2007–2008

Results Portfolio 4
Small Grants Scheme

World Health Organization
Regional Office for the Eastern Mediterranean

WHO Library Cataloguing in Publication Data

World Health Organization. Regional Office for the Eastern Mediterranean

Operational research in tropical and other communicable diseases: final report summaries 2007-2008: results portfolio 4 small grants scheme / WHO Regional Office for the Eastern Mediterranean

p.

1. Communicable Disease Control 2. Tropical Medicine - prevention and control 3. National Health Programs 4. Research 5. Vaccines 6. Case Reports I. Title II Regional Office for the Eastern Mediterranean
(ISBN: 978-92-9021-703-9) (NLM Classification: WC 680)
(ISBN: 978-92-9021-704-6) (online)

Design by Madiha Sandhu

Printed by Metropole, Egypt

Contents

Foreword

In the name of God, the Compassionate, the Merciful

It is increasingly recognized that poor health hinders human and economic development. Today, communicable diseases account for 50% of the burden of disease of developing countries. This is all the more striking when one considers that 80% of the world's population lives in developing countries. The control of infectious diseases is thus fundamental for poverty alleviation, and especially in disease-endemic countries. Of key relevance is the urgent need to push for research aimed at developing more effective tools and strategies to fight the infectious diseases of the poor. Building research capacity and leadership in developing countries themselves is increasingly seen as a critical component of this effort, and as a means to support human and economic development.

In order to break the vicious cycle of poverty and disease, WHO has developed a new strategy on research for health and is working on the mobilization of resources to implement this strategy. This strategy will be adapted at the regional level in 2010. The main objective of the strategy is the use of research results to reduce disease burden. It also aims at strengthening the research capacity in disease-endemic countries. This is essential as the evidence of the association between research and development in general, and health development in particular, becomes stronger and more compelling each year.

This is the 4th portfolio of operational research activities for communicable diseases supported by WHO Regional Office for the Eastern Mediterranean. The aim of the publication of these final report summaries is the documentation and dissemination of research findings for their effective use in disease control. Throughout this series of portfolios, we, as WHO, have highlighted, the implications of these findings for disease control. This collection of summaries is no different. The implications and corresponding recommendations have been communicated to the countries as an outcome of the WHO-sponsored research. In parallel, we have monitored the extent of translation of these research findings into policy and practice in the national programmes, as well as the publications originating from these supported projects. The main challenge has been the need to develop a mechanism for monitoring these important indicators of the impact of WHO-supported research projects on disease control. This challenge is being addressed.

The publication of this portfolio is an opportunity to invite researchers and disease control programmes in the Region to use these findings for more effective disease control. I take this opportunity to invite them to communicate with us and inform us about their experience in using these research findings and their impact on policy and practice.

Hussein A.Gezairy MD FRCS
WHO Regional Director for the Eastern Mediterranean

Preface

The WHO Regional Office for the Eastern Mediterranean supports operational research in tropical and other diseases through the TDR Small Grants Scheme. The scheme encourages collaboration between national control programmes and researchers from academia.

This publication summarizes each of the final reports of the research projects. The summaries include the key research results and their implications for disease control. However, this is not a peer reviewed publication and the investigators are encouraged to submit their manuscripts to indexed journals. This would provide evidence for the reliability of reported results with regard to the international scientific community. This issue includes an updated list of almost 100 articles resulting from Small Grant Scheme-supported research published in indexed journals.

It is hoped that the research-driven and evidence-based recommendations reported in this issue will be used to improve programme performance, increase the access of the community to timely diagnosis and effective treatment, and assist national control programmes in achieving the UN Millennium Development Goals.

Avian influenza

Knowledge, attitudes and practice study and risk analysis of avian influenza: an intervention study in three governorates in Lower Egypt

- **Egypt**
  Lower Egypt
- **Study period**
  September 2006–August 2007

- **Small Grants Scheme**
  (SGS) 2006 No. 82

- **Principal Investigator**
  Taghreed Farahat
  Faculty of Medicine
  Shebin El Kom City,
  Menoufia Governorate, Egypt
  e-mail: taghreedmfarahat@yahoo.co.uk

Abstract

Avian influenza is an infectious viral disease of birds caused by a type "A" strain of the influenza virus. This strain of influenza A (H5N1) is now spreading from birds, chicken, ducks and turkeys to humans. The objective of the study was to assess knowledge, attitudes, practice and risky behaviour of farm workers, the community, veterinaries and health-care workers regarding avian influenza infection in the three Egyptian governorates that reported the highest rates of infection.

Results Except for veterinaries, the level of knowledge of the studied groups was generally suboptimal. Adherence to protective measures was incomplete as a result of inadequate knowledge and negative attitudes towards avian influenza. Female gender, age less than 10 years, living in the Nile valley, and winter and spring seasons were significant risk factors for acquiring infection. The majority of target poultry was not vaccinated. Many challenges face control programmes, including risky behaviour of the community and farm workers, the cultural and geographical nature of Egypt, the relative shortage in funding and inadequate veterinary manpower.

Conclusion Defective knowledge and negative attitude towards avian influenza among the community, health-care and farm workers are factors threatening the spread of the disease. Raising awareness and comprehensive control measures are urgently needed.

Background

An outbreak of avian influenza caused by a strain of H5N1 occurred in Asia in the autumn of 2003 and spread in domestic poultry farms at a historically unprecedented rate. The outbreak tapered off in spring 2004 but in summer re-emerged in several countries in Asia. In the summer of 2005, H5N1 began expanding its geographic range beyond Asia; this trend has continued into 2007. There is particular cause for concern because this strain of influenza A (H5N1) is now spreading from birds, chicken, ducks and turkeys to humans, and scientists are trying to determine if the virus is also spreading from human to human. Avian influenza or bird flu presents a real possibility of a pandemic. The ongoing outbreak of avian influenza in poultry in Egypt and the reported human cases have generated much interest and concern in the region.

Materials and methods

The Menoufia, Gharbia and Kafr El-Sheikh governorates were selected due to their high prevalence of avian influenza among poultry and the detection of human cases. One quarter of the farms from each governorate were selected randomly. Poultry workers in the selected farms who were present at the study time and who agreed to be involved in the study were enrolled. All veterinaries who were present in the veterinary

Conclusions and implications of the study

- Raising awareness and improving community health-related literacy as well as capacity building of health workers, veterinaries and farm personnel are key interventions towards controlling avian influenza outbreaks in the community.
- Veterinaries, health-care and farm workers expressed negative attitudes by reporting that they were not prepared to buy protective clothes; however, if these clothes were distributed free, they were willing to use them. This economic situation should be appropriately handled to improve behaviour among these high-risk groups.
- Outbreaks of avian influenza in poultry cause devastating economic losses as they are generally controlled through extensive culling of infected birds. Vaccination of poultry is the most cost-effective measures in any avian influenza control programme. Vaccination should target farm poultry as well as domestic birds.
- Increased licensing of sanitary slaughter houses in all governorates would support the control of avian influenza.
- The capacity for country and regional surveillance should be strengthened and interministerial committees should be set up for rapid flow of information. Well-established mechanisms for regional networking and information sharing during control efforts are essential.

unit at the time of the study and who agreed to take part in the study were enrolled. The target groups in the selected districts were the farm workers, community members, veterinarians and health-care workers. These were given a knowledge, attitude, practice and behaviour (KAPB) questionnaire and an intervention by a health education programme. Tools of the study included predesigned questionnaire sheets to collect data related to KAPB in the four study groups regarding avian influenza and also a checklist to monitor the daily pattern of behaviour of workers and their use of personal protective clothing and equipment.

Main study findings

Among the studied health-care workers, 50%–60% were found to have correct knowledge about avian influenza. More than 85% of these knowledgeable health-care workers had gained their knowledge through Ministry of Health activities; however, they were not fully aware about the national plan against avian influenza, or the correct treatment and places for health care of patients with avian influenza. Nearly one half of all health-care workers acknowledged breeding birds at home and allowing children to play with them. Unsanitary disposal of poultry wastage and lack of vaccination were among their risky behaviours.

Among the farm workers studied, the majority (80–85%) gave unsatisfactory answers regarding correct methods of transmission of the disease. They did not adhere to wearing protective clothing and handled poultry disposal in unhygienic ways.

The majority of the veterinaries had satisfactory knowledge about avian influenza. They expressed a negative attitude by reporting that they were not prepared to buy protective clothing due to economic constraints. However, they would be willing to use protective clothing if this was distributed freely.

The community household participants showed poor knowledge regarding avian influenza. They expressed their panic but 80% continued to buy and consume poultry and eggs. Poor knowledge and negative attitude resulted in poor practices in two thirds of the studied community. Female gender, age less than 10 years, living in the Nile valley, and winter and spring seasons were identified as risk factors for avian influenza.

Although the target poultry population to be vaccinated was estimated at 150 million, only 60 million were covered by vaccination. Challenges facing avian influenza control were related to the behaviour of the community and farm workers and owners, the geographical nature of Egypt, relatively inadequate funding and insufficient veterinary manpower.

Conclusions and recommendations

The level of knowledge regarding methods of transmission and prevention was inadequate among the studied population. Risk factors included female gender, age less than 10 years, season, geographical residence, community and farm-workers' behaviour, inadequate funding and the shortage of veterinaries. These factors should be addressed to increase the efficiency of control measures and improve preparedness for future outbreaks of avian influenza.

Cutaneous leishmaniasis

Evaluation of integrated pest management in the control of zoonotic cutaneous leishmaniasis, Islamic Republic of Iran

- **Islamic Republic of Iran**
  Natanz county
- **Study period**
  January 2006–October 2007

- **Small Grants Scheme**
  (SGS) 2006 No. 2

- **Principal Investigator**
  Mohammas Motovali Emami
  Kerman University
  Isfahan, Islamic Republic of Iran
  e-mail: mtvimm@yahoo.com

Abstract

A study was conducted to evaluate integrated pest management (IPM) in the control of cutaneous leishmaniasis. Integrated management activities included the use of long-lasting insecticide-treated nets, rodent-control operations, residual spraying and environmental sanitation.

Results Of 12 624 persons who entered the area from non-endemic regions, 702 persons (5.6%) were infected. From May 2006 to November 2007 (during and after the intervention), 80 129 persons were enrolled in the study, 59 712 of them lived in other leishmaniasis foci. From the remaining 20 417, 31 (0.1%) patients with cutaneous leishmaniasis were detected. Results of 20 isolates showed that the parasite from human indigenous cases was *Leishmania major*.

An area of 410 ha around Emamzadeh Agha Ali Abbas was treated for rodent control. The total number of rodent holes was 36 059 (about 88 holes/ha). Rodent-control intervention resulted in an 85.6% decrease in rodent holes. A total of 4711 adult sand flies were collected from April 2006 to October 2007, 4602 of these were from rodent burrows and 109 were from indoor resting places in rooms in Emamzadeh. *Phlebotomus papatasi* (86.1%) and *Sergentomyia sintoni* (13.9%) were found in the rooms, while *P. papatasi* (23.9%), *P. sergenti* (1%), *P. caucasicus* (0.5%), *P. alexandri* (0.07%), *P. major* (0.3%) and *S. sintoni* (74.3%) were collected. in the rodent burrows.

Conclusion IPM is an effective and suitable means of preventing and controlling zoonotic cutaneous leishmaniasis (ZCL). The incidence of ZCL after the intervention was considerably less than before the IPM.

Background

Natanz county in Isfahan province, central Islamic Republic of Iran is well known for its hyperendemicity for zoonotic cutaneous leishmaniasis (ZCL). Many methods have been employed separately for the control of ZCL in Isfahan province, for example the use of residual insecticides indoors [dichloro-diphenyl-trichloroethane (DDT) 75% (2 g/m^2)], the use of DDT in rodent burrows or eradication of rodents within a 300-m distance of households; however, these methods have not been successful in disease control.

Integrated pest management (IPM) seeks to improve the efficacy, cost effectiveness, ecological soundness and sustainability of disease-vector control. In view of the high endemicity of ZCL in Isfahan province and the limited application of control measures, the present study was carried out to assess the efficacy of integrated control methods on minimizing ZCL in a contained area. These measures included control of rodents by baiting, control of sand flies by residual insecticides, environmental sanitation and the use of insecticide-treated bednets, in combination with health education and promotion.

Materials and methods

Natanz county in Isfahan province, central Islamic Republic of Iran is well known for its hyperendemicity for zoonotic cutaneous leishmaniasis (ZCL). Many methods have been employed separately for the control of ZCL in Isfahan province, for example the use of residual insecticides indoors [dichloro-diphenyl-trichloroethane (DDT) 75% (2 g/m^2)], the use of DDT in rodent burrows or eradication

Conclusions and implications of the study

- IPM entails the use of a range of interventions of proven efficacy, either separately or in combination, in order to implement more cost-effective control and reduce reliance on any single intervention.
- The use of long-lasting insecticide treated nets (Olyset® nets), rodent-control operations, residual spraying and environmental sanitation can provide protection from sand fly bites and thus interrupt transmission of ZCL.
- An IPM approach takes into account the available health infrastructure and resources and integrates all available and effective measures, whether chemical, biological or environmental.
- IPM also encourages effective coordination of the control activities of all sectors that have an impact on vector-borne diseases.
- The engagement of communities is a key factor in assuring sustainability of IPM.

of rodents within a 300-m distance of households; however, these methods methods have not been successful in disease control.

Integrated pest management (IPM) seeks to improve the efficacy, cost effectiveness, ecological soundness and sustainability of disease-vector control. In view of the high endemicity of ZCL in Isfahan province and the limited application of control measures, the present study was carried out to assess the efficacy of integrated control methods on minimizing ZCL in a contained area. These measures included control of rodents by baiting, control of sand flies by residual insecticides, environmental sanitation and the use of insecticide-treated bednets, in combination with health education and promotion.

Main study findings

Of 12 624 persons from non-endemic regions entering this area, 702 persons (5.6%) were infected. From May 2006 to November 2007 (during and after the intervention), 80 129 persons were visited, 59 712 of them lived in other leishmaniasis foci. From the remaining 20 417 person, 31 (0.1%) patients with cutaneous leishmaniasis were detected. Examination of 20 isolates from human indigenous cases identified the parasite as *Leishmania major*.

An area of 410 ha around Emamzadeh Agha Ali Abbas was treated for rodent control. The total number of rodent holes was 36 059 (about 88 holes/ha). These holes were closed and 7193 (about 18 holes/ha) were reopened before the first baiting in May 2006. The number of rodent holes decreased to 4019 (about 10 holes/ha) in August 2006, the second stage of baiting. The number of holes then decreased to 1525 (about 4 holes/ha) in November 2006, further decreasing to 1031 (about 2 holes/ha) in October 2007, 17 months after the first baiting. These results showed a 85.6% decrease of rodent holes.

Of the rodents caught around the Emamzadeh area, five *Rhombomys opimus* were infected with *Leishmania* in one or both ears, although most had no obvious cutaneous lesions. Polymerase chain reaction (PCR) examination confirmed the isolated parasite to be *L. major*.

From April 2006 to October 2007, a total of 4711 adult sand flies were collected and identified, 4602 from rodent burrows and 109 from indoor resting places in rooms in Emamzadeh. *Phlebotomus papatasi* (86.1%) and *Sergentomyia sintoni* (13.9%) were found in the rooms, while *P. papatasi* (23.9%), *P. sergenti* (1%), *P. caucasicus* (0.5%), *P. alexandri* (0.07%), *P. major* (0.3%) and *S. sintoni* (74.3%) were collected from the rodent burrows. The sand flies started to appear in mid-April and had disappeared by November. No sand flies were found in the area from December 2006 to April 2007. Dissection showed that 9.25% of *P. papatasi* (37/400) were infected with leptomonads.

Conclusions and recommendations

The incidence of ZCL considerably decreased after these interventions, thus IPM is an effective and suitable means of preventing and controlling ZCL. Through evidence-based decision-making, IPM rationalizes the use of human and financial resources and organizational structures for the control of vector-borne disease and emphasizes the engagement of communities to ensure sustainability.

Yemen

Diarrhoeal diseases

Effect of zinc supplementation on morbidity due to diarrhoea in infants and children in Elsabeen Hospital in Sana'a, Yemen

- **Yemen**
  Baher El Jabel State
- **Study period**
  2005–2006
- **Small Grants Scheme**
  (SGS) 2005 No. 37

- **Principal Investigator**
  Muna Abdo Mohammed ElNemr
  The University of Science and Technology Elseteen, Boys Campus
  Sana'a, Yemen
  e-mail: munaabdo@hotmail.com

Abstract

A study was conducted in Yemen to evaluate the effect of zinc supplementation on the mortality and morbidity of children with acute diarrhoeal illness under the age of 5 years. A total of 180 children, aged 3 months to 2 years, presenting with acute diarrhoea to the oral rehydration therapy centre in Elsabeen Teaching Hospital in Sana'a were admitted to the medical ward. They were then enrolled in a double-blind, case–control study where, after informed consent from the parents, one group received zinc sulphate for 14 days and were then followed for 2 months.

Results Children in the zinc-receiving group had fewer diarrhoeal episodes and a reduced volume of stools during hospitalization and during the follow-up period. Moreover, zinc was palatable to a significant degree.

Conclusion This study showed that administration of zinc for 2 weeks during acute diarrhoeal episodes could decrease the incidence of further diarrhoeal episodes, as well as decreasing the severity of these episodes.

Background

Diarrhoea represents a leading cause of death in children less than 5 years of age in the developing countries and in many countries of the Eastern Mediterranean Region, including Yemen. WHO estimates overall under-5 mortality to be 113/100 000 live births, of which diarrhoea accounts for 17%, while measles represents only 4% and malaria 3%. Hence, reducing the burden of diarrhoea in these countries will reduce the overall mortality. Zinc deficiency is highly prevalent in children in developing countries. Diarrhoea causes further loss of zinc in the stools, thus zinc deficiency is exacerbated in children with acute diarrhoea. Provision of zinc during diarrhoea is thus rationalized. Given the high prevalence of micronutrient deficiencies and infectious diseases in children of developing countries, interventions to reduce infant and preschool morbidity are a public-health priority. Since both diarrhoea and zinc deficiency are prevalent in developing countries, our hypothesis was that zinc supplementation during diarrhoea will reduce the frequency of subsequent attacks and their duration and severity.

Conclusions and implications of the study

- Zinc supplementation substantially reduced the incidence of severe diarrhoea and frequency of motions, the two important determinants of diarrhoea-related mortality and malnutrition.
- This intervention also substantially reduced the proportion of children who experienced recurrent diarrhoea. The effects are large enough to merit routine use of zinc during acute diarrhoea in developing countries. Prompt measures to improve zinc status of deficient populations are warranted.
- Potential approaches to achieve this goal include food fortification, dietary diversification, cultivation of plants that are zinc dense or have a decreased concentration of zinc-absorption inhibitors, and supplementation of selected groups of children.
- Future studies should assess the impact of increased zinc intakes on childhood mortality in developing countries. To facilitating intervention, reliable estimates of zinc deficiency are required, particularly in developing countries. In addition, the effects of longer periods of zinc administration after the initial attack should be studied, for example 3–4 months of daily zinc.

Materials and methods

This was a double-blind, randomized, placebo-controlled prospective clinical trial. After informed consent from the parents, 180 children with acute diarrhoea were randomly assigned into two treatment groups. One group received zinc acetate 20 mg/day (Indimedica Pharmaceuticals, India) daily for 14 days. The other group received identical placebo bottles. Children in both groups were offered oral rehydration therapy and parents were advised how to use it. Both groups were followed-up for the following 2 months.

Personal data were recorded for both groups. Children were followed by observing the date of the first episode, its duration, frequency of stools, acceptability, adherence to the treatment, as well as the number of episodes, amount and frequency of stools in each episode, duration of hospital stay, if any, and death and its cause, if any.

Main study findings

A total of 180 children were enrolled, 92 in the control group and 88 in the intervention group. There were no statistically significant differences among children in the groups with regard to age, gender, weight and height. The mean number of episodes during the follow-up period, mean frequency of stools in these attacks, and mean duration of hospital stay were significantly reduced in children receiving zinc during follow-up.

Conclusions and recommendations

The study showed that administration of zinc for 2 weeks during acute diarrhoeal episodes decreased the incidence of further diarrhoeal episodes, as well as the severity of these episodes.

Diarrhoeal diseases

The impact of LifeStraw® in reducing the burden of diarrhoeal diseases in Elmasraf settlement camp, south Gezira, Gezira State, Sudan

- **Sudan**
  Gezira State
- **Study period**
  September 2006–June 2007

- **Small Grants Scheme**
  (SGS) 2005 No. 136

- **Principal Investigator**
  Salwa Elsanousi Hussein
  Faculty of Medicine
  University of Gezira
  Wad Medani, Gezira State
  Sudan
  e-mail: salwasanousi@yahoo.com

Abstract

A study was conducted to test the use of LifeStraw® water purifiers for provision of safe water in Elmasraf camp, Gezira State, central Sudan during September 2006 to June 2007. The aims of this study were to assess the effectiveness of LifeStraw® in reducing the incidence of diarrhoea in the study population, to determine the acceptance of the community to its use and to test the efficacy of the device in purifying and treating canal water.

The study design was a prospective interventional surveillance including LifeStraw® provision and utilization. The targeted group was residents of Elmasraf camp who were 2 years of age and above, and who had consented to participate in the study. A preintervention survey showed that the incidence of diarrhoea was 16.8%.

Results The study revealed a significant reduction in the incidence of diarrhoea from 16.8% to 2.3% ($P < 0.0001$). The number of diarrhoeal episodes markedly reduced from 109 (in the preintervention survey) to 14 in the postintervention survey. The LifeStraw® device was readily accepted by the study population and was even requested by the residents of nearby camps who were not originally included in the study. Regular users of LifeStraw® understood its benefits in reducing diarrhoea episodes, while non-regular users claimed difficulty of use as the main factor. Analysis carried out at the Gezira State Water Corporation central laboratory showed that coliform bacilli count was significantly reduced after passing canal water through LifeStraw®.

Conclusion LifeStraw® is effective in purifying contaminated drinking water and reducing the incidence of diarrhoea. The device was readily accepted by the study population.

Background

At any given moment, about half of the world's poor are suffering from waterborne diseases, of which over 6000, mainly children, die each day by consuming unsafe drinking water. Today, more than 1 billion people are without access to safe water. Diarrhoea remains a leading cause of morbidity and mortality in Sudan, particularly among children. Gezira State is the second most populous state in Sudan (population 3.9 million), 79% of whom live in rural areas that include 1170 camps (campo) scattered around the Gezira scheme canals, where populations from different regions and ethnic groups come to work as agricultural workers. Gezira State includes seven localities, three of which include canal-irrigated agricultural projects. More than half a million in Gezira State (about 12.5%) are living in camps around the Gezira scheme; the majority of them have no access to safe water. The only source of drinking water in these camps is directly from the canals. Some of the camps have water hand pumps. The selected locality of this study was south Gezira, which has a population of 613 667. There are 252 camps in this area, about 50% of which have no access to safe drinking water.

LifeStraw® offers relief from waterborne diseases of major public-health concern, such as typhoid, cholera, dysentery and diarrhoea. It is a portable water-purification tool that is just 25 cm long and 29 mm in diameter and can be hung around the neck. LifeStraw® requires no electrical power or spare parts. It filters a minimum of 700 litres of water and effectively removes most of the microorganisms responsible for causing waterborne diseases, killing and removing 99.999% of waterborne bacteria, 99% of waterborne viruses and removing particles down to 15 μm. It is designed to turn

Conclusions and implications of the study

- LifeStraw® is effective in purifying contaminated drinking water and reducing the incidence of diarrhoea.
- The device was readily accepted by the study population as it was easy to carry and easy to use.
- As the burden of diarrhoea is mainly in infancy, the device should be modified in such a way that infants can also benefit from it.

surface water into drinking water, thus providing access to safe water with minimum cost.

The aim of the study was to assess the effectiveness of LifeStraw® in reducing the incidence of diarrhoea; to determine the acceptance of its use by the study population in the study population at Al-Masraf camp, Gezira State, Sudan; and to test the efficacy of the purification device in reducing the microbial content of canal water.

Materials and methods

The study was conducted in south Gezira, Gezira State, which has a population of 613 667 in 252 camps. About 70% of the camps have no access to safe drinking water. Permanent residents of El-Masarf camp who were more than 2 years of age and who consented to participate were included in this study. Of 134 households, 647 individuals were eligible. This was a prospective interventional surveillance design, through which LifeStraw® was used as an intervention. There were three phases.

In phase one (preintervention, from 22 September to the end of October 2006), a household survey was conducted by a trained team using pretested and modified questionnaires and an observation checklist. Subjects who had diarrhoea 2 weeks prior to the study were treated and followed for 4 months, to report and manage any new episodes of diarrhoea.

In phase two (intervention, from October 2006 to June 2007), participating residents were provided with LifeStraw® and trained in its use. Residents were closely monitored and followed to determine the incidence of diarrhoea. Throughout the study period, diarrhoeal episodes were reported, investigated and treated.

In phase three (post-intervention, from August 2006 to June 2007), post-intervention surveillance for the appearance of any diarrhoeal episode was carried out and a survey was performed using the same questionnaire as used in the preliminary survey. In addition, questions about the use of, and compliance with, LifeStraw® were included.

Well-structured pretested questionnaires for pre- and post-intervention surveys and observation checklist were designed to record sociodemographic characteristics, any history of diarrhoea or other waterborne diseases in the weeks prior to the survey, investigations carried out and the treatment given for these diseases. The observation checklist was used for recording household environmental condition, food and personal hygiene. In the post-intervention questionnaire, compliance with using LifeStraw® and desire to use the device in the future was recorded. The data were collected by a team of seven highly trained students from the University of Gezira, a medical assistant, two laboratory technicians, seven community supervisors with field experience and two medical officers, who were also field managers.

Collected stool specimens were sent for analysis, culture and sensitivity at the laboratory. Samples obtained from canal water were tested for bacterial content by the Gezira State Water Corporation central laboratory before and after passing through LifeStraw®.

Main study findings

The total number of households in Elmasraf camp was 134 and the total number of subjects included in the preliminary survey was 647, half of whom were male. Age distribution analysis of the study population revealed the highest percentage was between 2 and 14 years of age (41.8%) and two thirds of the study population was under 24 years of age. Almost two thirds (64%) were illiterate, one fifth (20%) were literate, while the remaining 16% were below school age. The only source of drinking water for more than three quarters of the study population at Elmasraf camp was from canals. Environmental conditions were poor in almost all households observed and personal hygiene and food safety were below standard.

The majority of the respondents (89%) who had diarrhoea in the preintervention phase belonged to a family of more than six. More than half the diarrhoeal episodes (51%) occurred in children 2–14 years of age and two thirds (67%) of the episodes occurred in those under 24 years of age. There was more than a threefold reduction in the incidence of diarrhoea among the study group (647) at Elmasraf camp before and after the intervention. The incidence of diarrhoea decreased from 16.8% to 2.3% ($P < 0.0001$). The frequency of diarrhoeal motions was significantly higher ($P = 0.015$) and the duration of the diarrhoea episode was significantly longer in the preintervention survey ($P = 0.047$). There was no significant difference in the type of diarrhoea in the pre- and post-intervention periods.

Only 29.4% (32/109) of the stool specimens obtained preintervention and 14.3% (2/14) obtained post-intervention were examined. There was no significant difference regarding species found during laboratory stool analysis for the episodes of diarrhoea in the pre- and post-intervention surveys. *Giardia lamblia* cysts, *Schistosoma mansoni* ova and *Entamoeba histolytica* cysts were detected in 22%, 11% and 7% of the specimens collected during the preintervention survey, respectively. *Giardia lamblia* cysts, *Schistosoma mansoni* ova or *Taenia saginata* ova were detected in 3.5% of specimens collected in the post-intervention survey. In the 44 specimens collected, seven bacterial pathogens were isolated (16%); six of which were identified as *Shigella* species, and only one isolate was identified as non-typhoidal *Salmonella*. Sensitivity to ciprofloxacin, nalidixic acid, gentamicin, trimethoprim and tetracycline was 100%, 100%, 85.7%, 14.3% and 0 %, respectively. About 50% of the pre- and post-intervention diarrhoeal episodes were treated medically. The remaining episodes were either not treated or received local remedies.

The canal water sites where the camp population collected water for drinking and household consumptions were tested. Tests revealed uncountable coliform bacilli in all specimens, indicating high contamination. After passing the canal water through LifeStraw®, analysis carried out at the Gezira State Water Corporation central laboratory showed that the coliform bacilli count was significantly reduced.

A total of 87% of the study population of Elmasraf camp were permanent users of LifeStraw® while the remaining 13%

were either occasional users or non-users. Non-regular users claimed difficulty of use as the main factor.

At the end of the study period, the research team conducted a post-intervention focus-group discussion (four groups: mothers, youth groups and men) to determine to what extent the study population desired to buy LifeStraw® the following year; 97% said that they would buy it but 3% said they would not, as they did not like it. Most of the population mentioned that one reason they would buy LifeStraw® the following year was that it enabled them to drink canal water safely while working in the field.

Conclusions and recommendations

The efficacy of LifeStraw® in purifying canal water has been demonstrated. Coliform bacilli count was significantly reduced by passing canal water through LifeStraw®. The study revealed a significant reduction in the incidence of diarrhoea after using LifeStraw® and the study population readily accepted the device. LifeStraw® should be modified in such a way that infants could also benefit from it.

Diarrhoeal diseases

Water quality and improving hygienic practices of the rural community in the vicinity of Ramallah, West Bank, occupied Palestinian territory

- **Occupied Palestinian territory**
  West Bank
- **Study period**
  April 2006

- **Small Grants Scheme**
  (SGS) 2005 No. 47

- **Principal Investigator**
  Ziad Mimi
  Water Studies Institute
  Birzeit University, Birzeit
  West Bank
  Occupied Palestinian territory
  e-mail: zmimi@birzeit.edu

Abstract

The aim of the study was to increase community awareness at the household level about hygienic practices and water quality, in order to develop an effective programme to change hygiene-related behaviour in the occupied Palestinian territory. The study was conducted in two rural villages near the city of Ramallah in the West Bank. A total of 50 households were selected from the two villages; mothers/housewives from each household were interviewed before and after face-to-face health education and awareness sessions to evaluate their knowledge, attitude and practices in regard to hygienic practices and water use. Water samples were obtained and analysed for chemical and biological properties.

Results The study reported the responses of each household to a questionnaire both before and after the educational sessions and the results demonstrated a statistically significant increase in hand-washing and showering practices after these sessions. The physical characteristics of the water samples were: pH 7.4, temperature 21 °C and turbidity 5.4 NTU. The numbers of samples contaminated with total coliform, faecal coliform and *Pseudomonas aeruginosa* were 4, 8 and 5, respectively.

Conclusion The results point to evidence that the process of basic hygienic behavioural education in itself is sound and with sufficient time could yield results by changing behaviour in participant groups at the community level.

Background

Proper hygienic practices can greatly affect waterborne diseases in the community. Statistics from the Palestinian Hydrology Group (2005 data) showed that 3% of the people in Ramallah suffered from waterborne diseases, while diarrhoea and gastroenteritis represented 3.4% of deaths in children between the ages of 1 and 4 years. Therefore it is of great importance to try to reduce these waterborne diseases and thus reduce the morbidity and mortality rates in children, as well as in adults. With mothers/housewives being the most important people affecting overall house hygiene, the focus of the study was on improving their awareness of proper hygienic practices.

Materials and methods

The study targeted 50 mothers/housewives of different ages, resident in two villages near Ramallah. Both villages have water networks connected to the household but no sewer network. The people in both villages dispose of waste in cesspits. The villages have electricity and phone networks. The research randomly targeted houses that had water-tanks or wells. In September 2005, mothers/housewives in each of the 50 households were interviewed by well-trained personnel who had previous experience of public-health surveys. The women were given a well-designed questionnaire that had been

Conclusions and implications of the study

- Sustaining individual counselling and health education at the household level will be crucial in maintaining an increased level of awareness and in promoting a sustainable improvement in hygiene practices.
- Observation of hygienic practices such as hand-washing may reveal important information about the use of soap and washing practices, which could help tailor information according to personal needs.
- Good communication with local civic leaders and influential persons will help facilitate these educational activities.
- Involvement of governmental institutions would also substantially improve the impact of these counselling and educational services.
- The possibility should be explored of establishing projects with sufficient resources and expertise to develop water and sanitation infrastructure; expand community-based behaviour-centred programmes to promote improved hygiene practices at the community and household level; and to facilitate policy development and institutional strengthening at multiple governmental levels to promote these goals and objectives. These projects should also include sufficient provision for strategic operational research to support policy development.

developed to assess their knowledge, attitude and practices related to some hygienic practices such as hand-washing, showering and water-storage practices at the household. The responses to the questionnaire were recorded both before and after proper education, and samples were taken from the water source tank and cistern at each house. In April 2006, field workers conducted the second visit. They evaluated the mothers/housewives new knowledge and practices, and also whether any mother/housewife cleaned her roof water tank. Motivations for promoting best practices and also barriers to adopting best practices were investigated.

Main study findings

The findings that were recorded after the educational intervention compared with the findings before the intervention showed a statistically significant increase in the awareness of the mothers/housewives about proper hygiene, reflected in an increase in showering, hand-washing and cleaning habits along with improved knowledge of the causes of waterborne diarrhoeal diseases and the affect of good hygiene on these diseases.

Conclusions and recommendations

The results presented point to evidence that the process of basic hygienic behavioural education in itself is sound and that, with sufficient time, continuing to focus efforts on behaviour change with participant groups at the community level could yield results. The information provides a solid basis for developing effective programme interventions that will continue to improve hygiene practices as part of a healthy lifestyle.

Hepatitis

Prevalence of, and risk factors for, hepatitis B and C viral infections among barbers and their regular clients in Gharbia Governorate, Egypt

- **Egypt**
  Gharbia Governorate
- **Study period**
  December 2006–
  November 2007

- **Small Grants Scheme**
  (SGS) 2006 No. 147

- **Principal Investigator**
  Safynaz Shalaby
  Department of Public Health
  Faculty of Medicine
  Tanta University
  Tanta, Egypt
  e-mail: shalabys@gmail.com

Abstract

The objectives of the study were to determine prevalence of hepatitis B virus (HBV) and hepatitis C virus (HCV) infections among barbers and a sample of their clients in Gharbia Governorate and to assess their knowledge, attitude and practices towards viral hepatitis infection.

Results Hepatitis B surface antigen (HBsAg) was detected in 4.2% of barbers and 3.9% of clients. The prevalence of HBsAg in urban barbers and clients was three times higher than that in rural barbers. Anti-HCV antibodies were detected in 12.5% of the total sample. The polymerase chain reaction (PCR) test revealed a prevalence rate of 9.1% in both barbers and clients. The prevalence among rural subjects was higher than that of urban subjects (10.2% and 8.1%, respectively). The level of knowledge was high in the majority of the study subjects. However, knowledge regarding the presence of protective drugs and vaccines was rather low. They had positive attitude towards antiseptic use after shaving, safe injection and were willing to have periodic testing. The majority of barbers observed good practices during shaving and cutting hair.

Conclusion The job of barber appeared to be of no risk for acquiring viral hepatitis. This may be due to the relatively good knowledge, positive attitude, and good hygiene and practice demonstrated by the majority of the barbers studied.

Background

The highest hepatitis C virus (HCV) prevalence in the world occurs in Egypt, where the prevalence of infection increases steadily with age. High rates of infection are observed among all age groups, although there are regional differences in the average overall prevalence [1,2,3]. The prevalence ranged from 10% to 20% of the general population, the rural population showing a higher prevalence than urban. This difference was attributed to past infection and treatment of schistosomiasis [4]. Barbers' shops are places where hair cutting, shaving and hair styling for men are practised. Malpractice during the use of sharp instruments may present the hazard of bloodborne infections and cause serious health problems for both barbers and clients [5].The objectives of this study were to determine prevalence of both hepatitis B virus (HBV) and HCV among barbers and a sample of their clients in Gharbia Governorate, Egypt and to assess their knowledge, attitude and practices regarding viral hepatitis.

Materials and methods

This study was carried out during 2007 in Gharbia Governorate, one of the governorates of the Nile delta in Egypt. The study took place in two of the eight administrative areas of the governorate, where nine administratively related

Conclusions and implications of the study

- In the present study, the detected total prevalence of HBsAg was 4.06%, which is near the lower limit of the recorded national range.
- There was a higher prevalence of HCV infection among barbers and clients in rural areas compared with urban areas, which may be correlated with the difference in schistosomial infection rates in both regions.
- The level of knowledge of subjects was relatively high, especially regarding modes of virus transmission. However, there was a deficit of knowledge concerning the sequel of hepatitis. This may be partly related to the source of their information, as friends and relatives constituted the main source of information in half the studied population.
- Among the subjects studied, there was a positive attitude towards safe injections and the use of antiseptics; this was more prominent among clients than barbers. This could be a reflection of good practice of barbers during shaving.
- The majority of barber shops satisfied good hygienic conditions.
- The sample size for barbers was well chosen to be representative of all barbers in the studied areas. However, the sample size of clients was relatively smaller and may have been less representative of all clients. Therefore, one limitations of the study is that it may give a broader picture of the situation among clients.

villages were randomly selected. The study sample size was 616 (308 barbers and 308 clients). A block-sampling technique using a map was used. Data were collected using a predesigned questionnaire. Direct observation was also made of the place and practice of the barbers while they worked. A blood sample (5 ml) was taken from each study subject through vein puncture using a Vacutainer® device and tested for hepatitis B surface antigen (HBsAg) and HCV antibodies. Samples that were positive for HCV antibodies were confirmed by polymerase chain reaction (PCR) tests for virus particles. Confidentiality of collected data and results was ensured.

Main study findings

HBsAg was detected in 4.06% of the studied population (4.2% of barbers and 3.9% of clients). The prevalence of HBsAg in urban barbers and clients was three times higher than that in rural barbers. Anti-HCV antibodies were detected in 12.5%. The infection rate was highest in rural clients (13.6%), followed by rural barbers (12.3%), while the prevalence of infection was equal among urban barbers and their clients (11.8%). Detection of the HCV particles using the PCR test revealed similar figures among both barbers and clients (9.1%).

Level of knowledge regarding mode of transmission was high in the majority of the study subjects. However, knowledge of protective drugs and vaccine was rather low. A positive attitude towards antiseptic use after shaving and safe injection was found among 55.8% and 49.0% of barbers, respectively, compared with 70.5% and 66.9% of clients, respectively. It was also found that 70.5% and 47.1% of barbers would like to be tested for viral hepatitis and other bloodborne diseases, respectively. While 94.5% of barbers changed blades for each client, about 75% disinfected used instruments and 63% washed hands. A total of 52.8% of urban barbers wore protective clothes, especially gloves, but only 9.6% of rural ones did this. Regarding shaving practice of clients, the practice of urban clients was revealed to be better than that of rural clients. On observing barbers' shops and their practice during shaving, it was found that in general, the majority of shops were well equipped, clean and tidy.

Conclusions and recommendations

This study revealed an almost similar infection rate of HBV and HCV among the selected study subjects compared with that reported nationally. The prevalence of infection in barbers was also similar to that in the clients. The job of barber appeared to be of no risk for acquiring viral hepatitis.

References

[1] Alter MJ. Epidemiology of hepatitis C virus infection. *World Journal of Gastroenterology*, 2007, 13:2436–2441.

[2] Abdel-Aziz F et al. Hepatitis C virus (HCV) infection in a community in the Nile Delta: population description and HCV prevalence. *Hepatology*, 2000, 32:111–115.

[3] Medhat A et al. Hepatitis C in a community in Upper Egypt: risk factors for infection. *American Journal of Tropical Medicine and Hygiene*, 2002, 66:633–638.

[4] Angelico M et al. Chronic liver disease in the Alexandria governorate, Egypt: contribution of schistosomiasis and hepatitis virus infections. *Journal of Hepatology*, 2000, 32:172–174.

[5] Mariano A et al. Role of beauty treatment in the spread of parenterally transmitted hepatitis viruses in Italy. *Journal of Medical Virology*, 2004, 74:216–220.

Hepatitis

Prevalence and risk factors of hepatitis B and C among barbers and their regular clients in Hyderabad, Pakistan

- **Pakistan**
  Sindh Province
- **Study period**
  2006–2007

- **Small Grants Scheme**
  (SGS) 2006 No.65

- **Principal Investigator**
  Tufail Bhatti
  Medical Research Centre
  Liaquat University of Medical & Health Sciences (LUMHS)
  Sindh, Pakistan
  e-mail: dr_tufailbhattia@yahoo.com

Abstract

A cross-sectional study was conducted to determine the seroprevalence of hepatitis B virus (HBV) and hepatitis C virus (HCV) among barbers and their clients in Hyderabad, Sindh, Pakistan and to assess their knowledge, attitudes and practices regarding these two viruses and their mode of transmission. A close-ended and open-ended questionnaire was designed to collect data from 715 participants (186 barbers and 529 clients). After obtaining informed consent, blood samples were withdrawn and tested for HBV and HCV markers by chromatography, enzyme-linked immunosorbent assay (ELISA) and polymerase chain reaction (PCR).

Results Interviews were carried out in 111 barber shops and a total of 715 questionnaires were completed by barbers and their clients. The mean age of both barbers (n = 186) and clients (n = 529) was 28.47 (± 9.7) years. Clients were aware of HBV and HCV and their route of transmission but barbers were less aware about the viruses and their transmission. Half of the respondents in both groups had heard about hepatitis B vaccination but only 15% had received the vaccine. Sixty per cent (60%) of the barbers claimed that they disinfected their instruments between clients and 88.9% claimed that they always used new blades. However, during observation of actual practices, only 28% disinfected their instruments between clients and 62% used a new blade for each client.

The seroprevalence of HBV was 4.8% and 6.0% in barbers and clients, respectively, and the seroprevalence of HCV was 6.5% and 17.2% in barbers and clients, respectively.

Conclusion There is some awareness among barbers and clients about HBV and HCV but poor knowledge about their mode of transmission. This warrants conducting a health education campaign to increase awareness of HBV and HCV and the risk factors associated with their transmission and to implement interventions to prevent their spread in the country.

Background

Hepatitis B and C are the most common blood-borne viral infections worldwide and are rapidly emerging as major public-health problems. Hepatitis B virus (HBV) infection is a major concern for health-care personnel today. Globally, 2 billion people are infected with HBV, of which more than 350 million (i.e. 5% of the world's population) are chronic carriers. Annually, up to 1 million people die due to consequences of HBV infection, such as chronic hepatitis, cirrhosis and cancer; HBV accounts for 60–80% of primary liver cancer cases globally.

An estimated 170 million people, 3% of the world's population, are chronically infected with hepatitis C virus (HCV), with 3–4 million people newly infected each year. There is no vaccine or postexposure prophylaxis for HCV, so the focus of primary prevention efforts should be on safe blood supply, safe injection practices and decreasing the number of people who inject drugs.

Important factors contributing to HBV and HCV spread include unsafe use of therapeutic injections, blood transfusion, being shaved by a barber, tattooing, mother-to-child transmission and unsafe sexual practices. The sharing of razors by barbers has been identified as a key risk factor for HBV spread in Italy, and sharing razors has also been responsible for HCV spread among psychiatric patients in Egypt, Japan and Pakistan.

Chronic HBV and HCV are major problems in Pakistan. Recent seroprevalence studies have demonstrated that 31% of the population have hepatitis B core antibodies, 4.3% have hepatitis B surface antigen, 6.5% have seroprevalence of HCV and 29% of chronic liver disease cases and 8% of liver cancer cases are seropositive. The spread of HBV and HCV in

Conclusions and implications of the study

- There is some awareness among barbers and clients about HBV and HCV but there is poor knowledge about their mode of transmission.
- Adequately disinfecting shaving instruments using antiseptic, and using new blades for every client instead of reusing blades, are extremely important practices and are highly recommended to limit the spread of HBV and HCV.
- Promoting health education campaigns to increase awareness among barbers about blood-borne viruses, in particular HBV and HCV, and the mode and risk factors associated with their transmission is crucial in preventing infection.

Pakistan is mainly due to blood transfusion and therapeutic injections. However, the excessive use of barbers for facial and armpit shaving is another risk factor for transmission. Little is known about the spread of blood-borne pathogens and the practices of barbers from Pakistan. Therefore, the purpose of this study was to determine the knowledge, attitudes, practices and risk factors of barbers of Hyderabad in order to implement measures to prevent HBV and HCV transmission among this high-risk group.

Materials and methods

A cross-sectional study was conducted from May to September 2007 in Hyderabad, Sindh province, Pakistan, which has an estimated population 28 914 880 (1998 census). A sample size of 715 (186 barbers and 529 clients) was therefore a reliable sample size for studying the prevalence of HBV and HCV as well as risk factors for acquiring infection. Sampling was carried out using a two-stage sampling technique. A close-ended and open-ended multicountry questionnaire was designed to collect data from participants. Blood samples were withdrawn after obtaining an informed consent and tested for HBV and HCV markers by chromatography, enzyme-linked immunosorbent assay (ELISA) and polymerase chain reaction (PCR).

Eligible participants were barbers who were involved in shaving, who had been working in a barber shop fore more than 1 year and who had consented to participate in the study, give a blood sample for testing and respond to the questionnaire. The information collected through the coded structured questionnaire, was processed and analysed.

Main study findings

The mean age of participants was 28.5 (± 97) years. The level of education was significantly higher among the clients, almost half of whom were professionals and were significantly more knowledgeable about HBV and HCV than the barbers.

More than 60% of clients but less than one third of barbers knew that sharing utensils, sexual contact, intravenous drug use, reusing needles, blood transfusion, dental procedures, scissors/surgical instruments, tattooing, barbers' shaving instruments and ear/body piercing are responsible for the transmission of both HBV and HCV.

Vaccine coverage for HBV was low among participants. Only 3% and 19% of participating barbers and clients, respectively, had received HBV vaccination.

Results of serum testing of the 715 blood samples by chromatography showed a 4.8% and 6.0% seroprevalence for HBV in barbers and clients, respectively, and a 6.5% and 17.2% seroprevalence for HCV in barbers and clients, respectively.

Regarding the attitudes of respondents, 88.9% of barbers claimed to use a new blade for each client. Also, 60% claimed to disinfect instruments between clients. However, during observation of actual practices, only 28% disinfected their instruments between clients and 62% used a new blade for each client.

More than three quarters of barbers shops were neat and clean and had electricity, about half the shops had adequate ventilation and 96% had ceiling fans. Only 30% of barber shops had good washing facilities.

Conclusions and recommendations

The general public and high-risk groups have inadequate knowledge regarding the modes of transmission, prevention and control measures of HBV and HCV. The study emphasized the need for health education campaigns about hepatitis. Strengthening infection-control measures in areas where a high risk of transmission is expected, such as in barbers, dental clinics and all health-care settings, is highly recommended.

HIV/AIDS

Factors affecting adherence of persons living with HIV to antiretroviral therapy in Lebanon

- **Lebanon**
  Nationwide
- **Study period**
  December 2005–December 2006
- **Small Grants Scheme**
  (SGS) 2005 No. 173

- **Principal Investigator**
  Eli Araaj
  Soins Infirmiers et Developpement Communautaire (SIDC)
  Beirut, Lebanon
  e-mail: sidc@lb.refer.org

Abstract

There are reports indicating the presence of barriers against optimal adherence to antiretroviral therapy (ART). A study was conducted to assess the personal, social and medical factors that affect the adherence of persons living with HIV (PLHIV) to ART. Seventy-two (72) patients were interviewed in three centres in Beirut [Soins Infirmiers et Developpement Communautaire (SIDC), Caritas and the Laboratory of Virology, Risk Hospital].

Results A total of 77.6% of the participants had taken ART for less than 10 years; of these, 38.8% had modified their ART regimen following their doctor's prescription. Of the total number of interviewees, 30.6% did not comply with their prescribed ART regimen. A total of 16.3% of participants reported interrupting their ART at least once. Of these participants who had interrupted their ART, 36.7% had done so for a period ranging from 1 day to more than 1 year, with unavailability of ART in the country being the main reason (61.1%). Factors affecting compliance with ART were social activity, having a close relationship, and educational level. The majority of participants expressed feelings of sadness and anxiety; however, their mental state did not affect compliance with ART.

Conclusion Factors affecting compliance with ART should be addressed and support should be given to patients to improve compliance.

Background

By the end of 2005, the cumulative total of reported HIV/AIDS cases in Lebanon was 903, with a male : female ratio 8:2. Of those, 318 were reported clinical AIDS cases [1]. Based on reports from the National Central Pharmacy, which is the supplier of government-subsidized antiretroviral therapy (ART), there are currently around 250 AIDS patients receiving ART in Lebanon [2]. ART was introduced into Lebanon in the early 1990s, with full government subsidy of triple therapy being introduced in 1996. Since then, frequent modifications of the drug distribution system have taken place in an attempt to remove barriers related to the availability of ART, improve confidentiality and patient anonymity, waiting time, inequity related to the different distribution mechanisms, reduce complication of procedures, etc. However, in the period preceding these modifications, several interruptions of therapy occurred, either due to drug unavailability or inaccessibility for the patients.

There is also reason to believe that persons living with HIV (PLHIV) in Lebanon have barriers against optimal adherence to ART. One study in Lebanon, conducted to assess stigma and discrimination in the context of HIV/AIDS, quotes patients talking about being embarrassed to take their medication in the presence of others, preferring to skip a dose when the presence of others was unavoidable [1].

Materials and methods

This study was a national cross-sectional study. Seventy-five (75) PLHIV in Lebanon were recruited through their physicians, support institutions and patient groups. Data

Conclusions and implications of the study

- The sample in this study reflected the national figures. The majority were male (84%) and a minority were female (16%). The group was aged between 20 and 59 years.
- The main mode of HIV transmission was sexual intercourse.
- Sixty-one per cent (61%) of participants gave the shortage of ART in the Central Pharmacy at the Ministry of Public Health as their main reason for interrupting their regimen..
- The study showed that belonging to a group of friends, having social activities and/or having a close relationship with one or more friends can be important factors in avoiding ART interruption.
- More than 71% of the participants had a very good impression of their health status.
- Interruption of ART regimen was not related to participants' feelings of sadness and anxiety. Moreover, 41% of participants found that their HIV status motivated them to be positive and active in their lives.

were collected using a questionnaire sheet that included the following information: sociodemographic data; treatment regimens used; patient's compliance with the prescription; support mechanisms available to patients; general health as perceived by the patient; patient's knowledge and attitude towards ART; patient's personal means of coping with stress and his/her general situation; and patient's assessment of his/her quality of life. Interviewers were recruited from the three different locations where the research was conducted (SIDC, Risk Hospital and Caritas). Interviewers were known and trusted by the PLHIV and had also been trained on data collection using the adopted questionnaire.

Main study findings

Among the interviewed PLHIV, 83.7% were males and 16.3% were females; 49% were aged between 20 and 39 years and 48.9% were aged between 40 and 59 years. The majority (63.3%) had been infected by unprotected sexual intercourse. A total of 77.6% of the interviewees had taken ART for less than 10 years; of these 38.8% had modified their ART regimen following their doctor's prescription. Concerning patient compliance with ART, 30.6% of the total number of interviewees did not comply with their prescribed regimen. A total of 16.3% of participants reported interrupting their ART at least once; of these, 36.7% had interrupted their ART for a period ranging from 1 day to more than 1 year, with unavailability of ART in the country given as the main reason (61.1%).

The need for support was expressed by 42.9%, who desired to belong to a group with whom they could share beliefs and decisions. Social activity and close relationships were found to affect adherence to ART. Concerning level of health, measured on a score from 0 to 10, 32.6% of interviewees ranked their health as being imperfect. Among participants with a lower academic level, 26.3% had interrupted their ART, representing the highest percentage of PLHIV who did so. The majority of the sample expressed feelings of sadness and anxiety (53%); although most of this group (61.5%) were disturbed by these feelings, no relationship was found between mental health status and adherence to ART. Living with HIV empowered and motivated 40.8% of interviewees to be positive and to find solutions to their situation in order to continue their normal life activities.

Conclusions and recommendations

Compliance with ART is crucial for the success of treatment and improving quality of life of PLHIV. Multiple factors affect the compliance of PLHIV and these should be identified and addressed by health-care workers, to ensure effectiveness of ART.

References

[1] *Adherence to long-term therapies: evidence for action.* Geneva, World Health Organization, 2003.

[2] National AIDS Control Programme. Beirut, Ministry of Health, 2004.

HIV/AIDS

Informal prostitution in Lahore: mapping its distribution, determinants and practices

- **Pakistan**
  Lahore
- **Study period**
  2006–2007
- **Small Grants Scheme**
  (SGS) 2006 No. 86

- **Principal Investigator**
  Shaheena Manzoor
  Institute of Public Health
  Lahore, Pakistan
  e-mail: prof_shaheena_Manzoor@hotmail.com

Abstract

A study was undertaken to provide information about the distribution, determinants and practices of informal prostitution in Lahore, Pakistan. The outcomes of the study may be used to aid HIV/AIDS prevention and awareness programmes for this high-risk population. The study was conducted in Lahore, which is the provincial capital and has a total population of 6 318 745. In-depth interviews were conducted with 83 subjects, selected by convenient sampling.

Results The mean age of the women was 26.14 years; 41% were married and another 28.9% were divorced or widowed. The majority (67.5%) had adopted the profession voluntarily without any violence or coercion; 46% said that no one in their family knew about their sex work while 23% said that people around knew about their sex work; 52% thought that sex work should be legalized and that brothels, escort agencies and other businesses related to adult prostitution should be licensed, with registered sex workers limited to certain areas and with mandatory health testing of the sex workers and their clients for HIV and other sexually transmitted infections.

Conclusion First sexual exposure and social environment determine a female's sexual way of life. Women sex workers are poor, uneducated, left by parents or husbands or, if living with them, may become sex workers to support ageing parents or husbands who may be out of work or drug addicts. Female prostitution is thus a manifestation of poverty.

Background

Unfortunately, despite hundreds of religious stalwarts and their organizations, policemen have proved helpless to stop "immoral trafficking", as they label this activity. According to a United Nations International Children's Fund (UNICEF) report, 55% of families from 35 localities in Lahore have one or more members as sex workers; the estimated total number of sex workers in the city is 55 000, with 19 000 of these child sex workers and the total number of households in Lahore involved in the sex trade is about 30 000. The aim of this study is to help improve conditions and rehabilitate women in the sex trade by highlighting their plight to policy-makers. The study focuses on factors that have been proposed as determinants of prostitution such as broken homes, marital stress and disharmony, easy money, emotional immaturity, international travel, tourism, social disruption and, above all. urbanization and industrialization.

Materials and methods

A cross-sectional community-based qualitative study was conducted in district Lahore, which is the provincial capital with a total population of 6 318 745. The study population is a mix of urban and rural communities. District Lahore is administratively divided into nine towns having 150 union councils. Total sample size was divided into nine groups, identified from different towns (clusters) of Lahore. Focused areas were the vicinities of theatres, cinemas, film studios, markets, public transport stands and the places known for the prostitution. Social mapping of the study subjects was carried out and subjects for interviews were selected with convenient sampling. In-depth interviews were conducted with 83 subjects.

Main study findings

Age ranged from 6 to 38 years, with mean age 26.14 years; 33.7% were in the age group 20–24 years. A total of 41% were married and another 28.9% were divorced or widowed. While many were illiterate (36.1%), 27.7% had reached primary

Conclusions and implications of the study

- Women involved in prostitution are a highly marginalized population who are rarely recognized as individuals with unique life histories. If we were able to explore the dimensions of these women's lives and better understand the issues behind the behaviour of prostitution, we could create a better match between what exists and what is needed, with the goal of treatment and prevention of risky behaviour.
- Initiation into multiple-partner sex may be by intimate relations with brothers-in-law and may ultimately lead young women into life as sex workers.
- Consequences of natural disasters such as earthquakes, which result in many deaths and disabilities, may also lead to misery in the lives of those women who escaped body injuries, especially young females.

level education. With respect to earnings, 47.7% earning more than 10 000 rupees per month, 27.7% earned from 5000 to 10 000 rupees while 9.6% were below the poverty line (i.e. US$ 2 per day). Regarding other occcupations, 3% of sex workers were solely engaged in sex work; the others were also working as domestic servants, jewellery makers, medical representatives, lady health visitors, nurses, office secretaries, telephone operators and tailors. A total of 70% were Muslim, while 15.5% were Christian.

A total of 65% of respondents had been in the profession for more than 3 years and 35% for more than 5 years; 30% of respondents used their homes for sex work; 9.6% picked-up their clients in the streets but a few were booked by telephone and performed sex in hotels, or in the homes or offices of their clients.

The majority (67.5%) said that they had adopted the profession voluntarily, i.e. without violence or coercion; however, 11% were forced circumstantially or through coercion. A total of 55.4% said that no one in the family knew about their sex work, while 27.7% were known sex worker. Of those, 43% said that behaviour of people towards them was sympathetic, while the remainder said they were discriminated against with people overtly or covertly expressing their hatred.

Regarding knowledge about modes of transmission of HIV/AIDS, 75%, 60%, 55% and 41% were aware of intimate sexual contact, sharing needles, blood transfusion and transmission from mother to child, respectively. The source of this information was friend/relative (57.8%), TV (42.1%) and health-care providers (34.9%). A total of 57% had no knowledge of safe sex; 85.5% reported using condoms during sexual acts with their clients but 70.4% used condoms sometimes or only if they remembered. Only 29.6% always used condoms. While 76.5% had active sex relations with their husbands, only 4 individuals always used a condom when having sex with their husbands.

A total of 51.8% reported smoking, 43.3% also used other substances but only 2 individuals were injecting; 20.5% had tattoos, only 29.41% of those with tattoos said that disposable needles had been used. Over a third (36.1%) had suffered from a sexually transmitted infection; 57% of these respondents had consulted a doctor. A total of 26.5% said that their health-care provider knew about their sex practices and 20.5% had taken a HIV test. Almost all (95%) respondents were unaware of any services available for them. However, 52% were of the view that sex work should be legalized, with licensing conditions for brothels, escort agencies and other businesses related to adult prostitution, limiting the sex work to certain areas, and with registration of sex workers, mandatory health testing of sex workers and their clients for HIV and other sexually transmitted infections.

Conclusions and recommendations

Women sex workers are poor, uneducated, having been left by parents or husbands or, if still living with them, having to work to support ailing parents or husbands who are out of work and are drug addicts. Female prostitution is a manifestation of the feminization of poverty.

Based on the findings of the study, we recommend the promotion of adult female education and information dissemination regarding the risks associated with sex work (i.e. promotion of safe sex). In addition we recommend the development of social support systems such as drop-in centres that would focus on basic needs such as food, clothing and shelter for abandoned women; promotion of vocational and life skills among women by establishing centres in slums and peri-urban areas; establishing health-care clinics in the vicinity of theatres and cinemas that would specifically address the needs of this population, including providing care and support for sexually transmitted infections and HIV, unplanned pregnancies, and injuries from physical and sexual violence. Community intervention is also required in order to establish safer areas in which women may prostitute in a "controlled" environment and to provide them with the same social benefits that are available to the rest of society, so that they can live safely and without prejudice and discrimination.

HIV/AIDS

Egypt

Evaluation of HIV voluntary counselling and testing services in Egypt

- **Egypt**
- **Study period**
  September 2006–September 2007
- **Small Grants Scheme**
  (SGS) 2006 No. 150

- **Principal Investigator**
  Ibrahim Kabbash
  Faculty of Medicine
  Tanta University
  Tanta, Egypt
  e-mail: iakabbash@hotmail.com

Abstract

The objectives of the study were to determine the level of satisfaction of service providers and clients of voluntary counselling and testing (VCT) centres and identify points of strength and weakness. All functioning VCT centres in Egypt were studied. The study sample consisted of 16 counsellors and 928 clients. Clients were interviewed to collect data using a predesigned questionnaire sheet. Counsellor data were collected through two focus group discussions.

Results The main motive for seeking VCT service was having had risky sexual behaviour (34.2%). More than 90% of clients reported satisfaction with the counselling service. Gender, educational level and the type of VCT centre significantly affected level of satisfaction. Only 41.4% were willing to discuss their test results with their partners. Problems highlighted by the service providers included the absence of a fixed job description, lack of administrative support, unsettled working rules and regulations, and lack of proper community awareness. Counsellors expressed the need for more training and an improved working environment, which would help to ensure privacy and confidentiality.

Conclusion The level of client satisfaction with the VCT services was generally high. To improve the quality of the service provided to clients, their problems should be highlighted and enabling factors reported, and the needs of counsellors should also be addressed.

Background

Knowing HIV infection status strengthens prevention efforts. HIV counselling and testing can lead to a reduction in the number of sexual partners, increased condom use, fewer sexually transmitted infections and safer injection practices [1]. Voluntary counselling and testing (VCT) in Egypt gives clients an opportunity to utilize anonymous pretest and post-test counselling services when considering an HIV test, and also links clients to a range of care and support services that meet their needs [2]. To improve quality of services provided, procedures for conducting VCT should be reviewed and updated regularly, in the context of national and/or situational changes related to HIV/AIDS in Egypt [3].

Materials and methods

The first VCT centre in Egypt was launched in January 2005. By the end of 2005, seven fixed and nine mobile centres distributed in different governorates of Egypt were providing VCT services. The study sample included 16 service providers at the studied VCT centres and 928 clients. The study utilized

Conclusions and implications of the study

- The present study revealed that the uptake of VCT services is low, especially in fixed centres, due to associated stigma with HIV/AIDS. The number of clients was higher in mobile centres as they also offer hepatitis B and C tests, which are needed by more people.
- The major barriers to HIV counselling and testing were having a VCT location that lacked privacy, along with issues of confidentiality and stigma problems. Other factors hindering uptake of services may be related to employment rules and regulations; management problems; clients/counsellor privacy and confidentiality; and general problems related to working with HIV.
- The majority of clients in the present study were males. Clients were mainly skilled workers. Females attended mobile centres significantly more often than fixed ones, which may reflect cultural trends with males accepting and desiring HIV testing more than females.
- The main motives for seeking VCT services were having had risky sexual behaviour, previous blood transfusion, and injecting drugs.
- Level of satisfaction of clients with VCT services was affected significantly by gender, higher education level, and among clients served by fixed centres.
- The majority of the clients studies reported satisfaction with the different stages of the counselling service and intended to tell others about the service. However, there was low intension to share test results with their partners.

qualitative and quantitative methods of data collection. A predesigned questionnaire was used to study the opinions of clients and service providers concerning their satisfaction with the provided service and positive and negative aspects of it. Data were collected through direct interviewing of study subjects. Two focus-group discussions were organized. The first focus group included counsellors from the fixed centres (six persons, two females and four males). The second focus group included counsellors from the mobile centres (nine persons, one female and eight males). Discussions were organized based on a previously prepared topic guide.

Main study findings

The total number of clients served by mobile centres was 28 310, which represented a rate of 262.1 clients served per month per centre. The rate of clients served by fixed centres was relatively much lower (33.1/month/centre). The majority of clients were in the age group 20–40 years (77.0%). More females used mobile centres (20.3%) than fixed ones (14.6%). Clients were mainly skilled workers (43.1%). Over two thirds of clients had secondary or university education (67.4%). The main motives for seeking VCT service were having had risky sexual behaviour (34.2%) and previous blood transfusions (22.3%). The main sources of information about VCT centres were relatives/friends (32.7%), posters/sign posts (24.5%), health-care workers (23.4%) and lectures (20%). More than 90% of clients reported satisfaction with the different stages of the counselling process. Only 57.9% of clients talked with their counsellor about previous or current HIV testing and only 41.4% were willing to share test results with their partners.

The majority of service providers were male (58%). Most service providers reported that they had received sufficient training, but still 66% reported the need for further training. Only 50% reported receiving enough incentives. the majority reported that their clients were in need of the service they provided, that their clients benefited from it and that their work helped to reduce HIV infection (98%, 100% and 100%, respectively). Eighty per cent (80%) of service providers felt comfortable serving clients with socially unacceptable behaviour and 82% reported that their clients accepted the concept of behaviour change. The majority of service providers in mobile centres complained of client overload (87.1%), while 68.4% of service providers in fixed centres complained of low rates of attendance among clients.

Conclusion and recommendations

Where VCT services are provided, the level of satisfaction of clients is generally high. Further interventions that may be required to improve the quality of the service provided include further training of service providers; providing a fixed job description and set working rules and regulations; more support for tackling administrative problems; improved community awareness and health education sessions; ensuring client privacy and confidentiality; and improving working environment, including addressing transport problems.

References

[1] *UNAIDS at country level: progress report.* Geneva, UNAIDS, 2004 (04.35E).

[2] *National guideline for voluntary counseling and testing.* Egypt, Ministry of Health and Population, Family Health International and USAID, 2004 (IMPACT project HRN-A-00-97-00017-00).

[3] Lamptey PR, Gayle HD. *HIV/AIDS prevention and care in resource-constrained settings.* Egypt, Family Health International and USAID, 2001 (project HRN-A-00-97-0017-00).

HIV/AIDS

The prevalence of transmitted HIV drug resistance in the Islamic Republic of Iran in 2005

- **Islamic Republic of Iran**
  Nine provinces
- **Study period**
  2005–2006
- **Small Grants Scheme**
  (SGS) 2005 No. 11

- **Principal Investigator**
  Sayed Mohesen Mousavi
  Center for Disease Control and Prevention
  Ministry of Health and Medical Education
  Tehran, Islamic Republic of Iran
  e-mail: smmousavi@yahoo.com

Abstract

A minimum-resource method called the HIV Drug Resistance Threshold Survey (HIVDR-TS) was used to estimate the prevalence of transmitted HIV drug resistance (HIVDR) in a newly infected, never-treated population in the Islamic Republic of Iran. The sources of the study population were Risk Behavior Consolation Centers in Tehran and in nine other provinces. Blood specimens from 73 infected individuals were sent for laboratory investigation at the National HIV and Retrovirology Laboratories, Public Health Agency of Canada (PHAC) to detect mutations known to be associated with resistance to drugs of the standard first-line regimens.

Results The mean age of participants was 20.9 ± 6.4 years, with a range of 14 months to 25 years. The majority of participants were male (67%), mostly of single marital status. The main mode of transmission was intravenous drug use (IDU) (64%), followed by heterosexual contact (22%). The mean duration of IDU was 4.4 ± 2.5 years. The specimen qualifications were perfect (50%), well (40%) and fair (10%). The mean length of dried blood spot (DBS) storage in refrigerators at 4–8 °C before shipping to the Center for Disease Control and Prevention (CDCP), was 1.5 ± 4.7 days, while the mean length of the DBS storage in freezers at -20 °C in CDCP was 93.2 ± 71.9 days before shipping to PHAC.

Conclusion It is feasible to study HIVDR before antiretroviral therapy (ART) is started to ensure success of the treatment regimen. Such information will also be helpful in evaluating the continued use of ART regimens.

Background

By the end of September 2006, the total number of individuals with HIV/AIDS registered by the Center for Disease Control and Prevention (CDCP) in the Islamic Republic of Iran was 13 702; intravenous drug use (IDU) was the main mode of transmission (64.6%). All injecting drug users were infected with HIV-1 subtype A. Thirteen prescriptions were presented in national guidelines for antiretroviral therapy (ART) but only four were routinely prescribed. In the Islamic Republic of Iran, ART was first used in 2003 in Tehran and Kirmanshah, and then later was used in other provinces. In 2005, the estimated number of individuals eligible for ART was 700–750. However, only 490 individuals are currently on ART. This number is estimated to be 900 by the end of 2007. There are no data on transmission of HIV/AIDS drug resistance (HIVDR). This study was designed to estimate the prevalence of transmitted-HIVDR in a newly infected, never-treated population in the Islamic Republic of Iran.

Conclusions and implications of the study

- Surveillance of drug resistance in a community may provide useful information for the design and selection of preferred ART drug combinations.
- Results can be used for evaluation of the continued utility of the HIV regimens in use, deliberations on whether baseline HIVDR testing before ART begins is feasible and desirable in certain settings, and as part of the evaluation of the ART programme success in minimizing the emergence and transmission of HIVDR.
- The numbers of eligible specimens were too few to use the WHO HIVDR threshold survey method to categorize the prevalence of transmitted drug-resistant HIV in any of the geographic areas surveyed. However, piloting the surveys in a number of areas supported an evaluation of methods and procedures in a variety of sites and geographic settings.
- Given the low prevalence of HIV in the general population, reaching the required sample size of 70 using the voluntary counselling and testing sites can be problematic. However, surveys focusing on IDU, using sites providing services to intravenous drug users, appear to be feasible.

Materials and methods

The study design was case series and a minimum-resource method called the HIV Drug Resistance Threshold Survey (HIVDR-TS) was used. A non-probability sampling (sequential sampling) method was used for site selection, based on the known or estimated extent of current or future availability of ART in various parts of the country. The sources of the study population were Risk Behavior Consultation Centers. All 10 of these centres in Tehran province and another nine centres from nine provinces (Esfahan, Fars, Hamadan, Kermanshah, Khozestan, Kordestan, Lorestan, Qom and Yazd) were selected for the study. Participants were women or men confirmed as HIV-positive who were under 25 years old, with no history of AIDS or of treatment for HIV/AIDS. Seventy-three (73) specimens were collected. Dried blood spots (DBS) were prepared and sent to the National HIV and Retrovirology Laboratories, Public Health Agency of Canada (PHAC) to detect any mutations known to be associated with resistance to drugs in standard first-line regimens. Resistance was considered by either the presence of at least one major mutation associated with resistance to one or more drugs in the standard first-line regimen, or a combination of other mutations. Prevalence of resistance was not estimated precisely, but rather was classified for each drug, or drug class, as < 5%, 5–15% and > 15%.

Main study findings

A total of 73 HIV-positive specimens were collected; however, two were deleted as they were from subjects over 25 years old. The mean age of participants was 20.9 ± 6.4 years, with a range of 14 months to 25 years; 67% of participants were male and 24% were female. The marriage rate was 13.7%, and 2.8% of those who had been married were divorced or widowed. A total of 31% were unemployed, 4.1% were uneducated and 64% were intravenous drug users. The mean duration of IDU was 4.4 ± 2.5 years. A history of heterosexual contact was reported by 22%, homosexual contact by 7%, blood transfusion by 7%, tattooing by 23%, and mother-to-infant transmission route was reported by 5.5%. The specimen qualification was perfect (50%), well (40%) and fair (10%). The mean length of the DBS storage in a refrigerator at 4–8 °C before shipping to CDCP was 1.5 ± 4.7 days, and the mean length of the DBS storage in a freezer at –20 °C in CDCP before shipping to PHAC was 93.2 ± 71.9 days.

Of the 73 specimens, 39 (53%) were amplified and sequenced. Of these, 18 eligible sequences came from eight different areas of the country; no more than four specimens were available from any one area. Threshold survey analyses to classify transmitted resistance could therefore not be performed. One eligible participant from Esfahan (ID 42) had a K219EQ reported in reverse transcriptase (RT); K219E appears on the WHO list of nucleoside RT inhibitor (NRTI) mutations associated with transmission of a drug-resistant strain. The sample quality of the associated specimen was reported as "poor". If a full analysis was being performed, PHAC would be asked to have a virologist confirm the presence of this mixture, and if its presence were confirmed, eligibility would be subsequently reviewed for this individual.

Two ineligible individuals also had sequences with relevant mutations. The first, a 25-year-old male from Esfahan (ID 43), had D67DG in RT; D67G appears on the WHO list of NRTI mutations associated with transmission of a drug-resistant strain. The sample quality for this specimen was reported as "perfect". The second, a 5-year-old female from Tehran (ID 23) had V75AV reported in RT; V75A appears on the WHO list of NRTI mutations associated with transmission of a drug-resistant strain. The sample quality for this specimen was reported as "poor". If these two individuals had been eligible and a full analysis was being performed, PHAC would be asked to review and confirm the presence of these mixtures.

Two atypical protease (PR) inhibitor mutations, I47M and G190R, appeared at resistance-associated positions in PR in the sequences of eligible participants 14 and 22, respectively. These mutations are not associated with transmitted resistance or any other kind of resistance. A common polymorphic mutation, V118I, appeared in the RT sequence of participant 65. This mutation appears naturally at levels > 2% in untreated populations with most HIV-1 subtypes and is not included on the WHO list of mutations associated with transmitted resistance.

Most PR sequences could be interpreted as HIV-1 subtype A, based on phylogenetic analyses. Some RT sequences were also interpretable as A, but most did not resemble any pure subtypes or acknowledged combination subtypes using either of these tools.

Conclusions and recommendations

Continued use of HIV drug regimens should be based on information regarding HIVDR. It is feasible to study HIVDR before ART commences, to ensure the success of the treatment regimen.

HIV/AIDS

Assessment of HIV/AIDS knowledge, attitudes and behaviour among university students in the Gaza Strip

- **Occupied Palestinian territory**
  Gaza Strip
- **Study period**
  November 2005 and June 2006
- **Small Grants Scheme**
  (SGS) 2005 No. 131
- **Principal Investigator**

Suliman Ebaid Eid
AMAN Programme for Sexual Health and AIDS
Lababidi Street, POB 1137
Occupied Palestinian territory
e-mail: amanproject@yahoo.com

Abstract

This study was carried out in the Gaza Strip and targeted university students. Eight hundred (800) students (53.1% males and 46.9% females) were randomly selected and then surveyed anonymously using a pretested questionnaire to assess their knowledge, attitude and behaviour towards HIV and AIDS.

Results Of 800 students surveyed, 97.3% had heard of HIV/AIDS and sexually transmitted diseases (STDs). The main source of information for males was the internet (61.5%), while the radio was the main source for females (41.3%). A total of 30.6% of students believed that condoms gave protection from HIV infection while 42.1% believed they did not; 56% thought that mosquitoes transferred the virus to humans and 20% believed that coughing or sneezing may spread the infection. Only 11.5% of males and 0.6% of females had been tested for HIV, although 51.4% had no objection to testing. Also, 45% of participants would refuse to share the same class as an HIV-infected person, 75% would not share food or drink and 28.4% would not shake hands with or kiss an HIV-positive person. They thought HIV-positive people practiced illegal sex, and 55.5% said they would only nominate them for a specific job or no job at all.

Conclusion Most of the participants knew about HIV and STDs but their knowledge was flawed. Stigma against people living with HIV affected youth attitude towards HIV-positive individuals.

Background

The first case of HIV/AIDS was reported in the Gaza Strip in 1986. Since then, special concern has focused on the surveillance of sexually transmitted diseases (STDs), including HIV/AIDS. Generally, the Gaza Strip has a low HIV/AIDS prevalence rate. The Ministry of Health is the main care provider for HIV/AIDS patients. Other health-care sectors will provide educational services to the targeted population when funds become available. There are no centralized or subcurriculum programmes available to meet university students' educational and behavioural needs. The Ministry of Health in the Gaza Strip faces problems in providing vital services to their different communities as a result of the conflict over the past decade; available resources are directed to meeting emergency and other vital care treatment. Since the prevalence of HIV/AIDS is very low and intervention is very expensive, HIV/AIDS does not fall within vital care. The aim of this study was to assess HIV/AIDS knowledge, attitudes and behaviour among university students in the Gaza Strip.

Materials and methods

The study was a cross-sectional survey with two additional focus-group discussion. The sample consisted of 800 randomly selected participants; one-half in their first year of study and the one-half in their fourth year. Of the two

Conclusions and implications of the study

- These results show a real gap between the knowledge and the attitudes and practices of the university students regarding HIV/AIDS.
- Owing to misconceptions about methods of transmission, there is a very strong stigma in the student community against HIV-positive individuals.
- It is important that policy-makers realize that school and university curricula may be the least-effective sources of information.
- New methods of transmitting information, such as short-message service (SMS) messaging on mobile phones have been neglected, in spite of them becoming very common methods of communication.
- A more open discussion of sexual issues among adolescents, adults and religious leaders would help to fight the common misconceptions associated with transmission of HIV as well as the stigma surrounding those with HIV.
- The Ministry of Health could play a strong role, not only in increasing awareness of HIV/AIDS but also in fighting the stigma associated with it, by providing dedicated voluntary counselling and testing units that would permitting anonymous testing. Such units could be established jointly with NGOs.

focus groups, one consisted of seven boys and the other consisted of seven girls. A questionnaire was designed and tested to cover: demography; knowledge regarding HIV and its transmission; control measures and prevention; attitudes toward the HIV-positive individual; attitudes towards risk behaviour; opinions on public policies and community beliefs; acceptance of HIV-testing polices; and acceptance of the voluntary counselling and testing programme. The focus groups also discussed three issues: available sources of information for HIV/AIDS; attitudes towards HIV-positive individuals; and whether more open public discussion should be encouraged concerning HIV/AIDS and related risk behaviour (sex and drugs).

Main study findings

The majority of the participants (97.3%) had heard about STDs and (95%) had heard about HIV/AIDS. Ten per cent (10%) considered AIDS to be a punishment from God and 69.2% rarely or never talked to their parents about AIDS. The main sources of information regarding AIDS were the internet for males (61.5%) and the radio for females (41.3%). Discussion of sexual health was mostly with religious leaders (77%); 70% believed that there was no contradiction between sexual health and religion. About 48% thought that HIV/AIDS was a problem in the occupied Palestinian territory.

The majority of participants were aware of the actual methods of HIV infection. However, there was some misconception about HIV transmission, including that the infection could be caught by kissing an HIV-positive person (30.1%), by sharing swimming pools (26.4%), from mosquitoes (49.5%) and by droplet infection (20%). Only 6.3% had been tested for HIV infection, although 51.4% were willing to have the test performed.

A total of 41.7% would refuse to share a classroom with an infected person and 63.4% would refuse to kiss an infected person. The majority (78.7%) also would refuse to share eating utensils with infected persons. The majority also said that they would stop dealing with a person known to be suffering from HIV, while 43.2% believed that such individuals should only be employed in specific jobs.

Conclusions and recommendations

The university students studied had inadequate knowledge of HIV and STDs. Their attitudes towards HIV-positive individuals need to be modified and more acceptance and consideration need to be shown to these persons as patients. Information should be distributed by concerned organization, especially the Ministry of Health, Ministry of Education and non-governmental organizations (NGOs). There is a need to initiate voluntary counselling and testing programmes with anonymous testing.

Infectious diseases

Study of prevalence of malaria, acute respiratory infection and diarrhoeal disease among children under 5 years of age in camps for internally displaced persons in Mogadishu, Somalia

- **Somalia**
  Mogadishu
- **Study period**
  January–December 2006
- **Small Grants Scheme**
  (SGS) 2006 No. 21
- **Principal Investigator**

Adan Haji Ibrahim Daud
Ala-Yasir Clinic
Mogadishu, Somalia
e-mail: dr_adan@hotmail.com

Abstract

Political turmoil and internal conflict resulting in severe fighting has led to mass displacement of the population in Somalia. Recurring pockets of conflict in different parts of Somalia has resulted in the constant movement of people and growing number of internally displaced person (IDP) settlements, especially in the south and central zones. There are 210 IDP camps scattered through Mogadishu's16 districts and more than 350 000 (14.3%) of the total population of Somalia live in these camps. The overall objective was to study the prevalence and determinants of malaria, diarrhoea and ARI in children less than 5 years in IDP camps in Mogadishu.

A cross-sectional observational surveillance study with nested case–control phase was conducted in Mogadishu IDP camps. The target population was children 6–59 months of age, or 65–110 cm, living in IDP camps. The sampling technique was a multistage cluster sampling technique.

Results Nine hundred (900) children were examined in Mogadishu IDP camps. Global and severe acute malnutrition was 15.4%. Of these malnourished children, 8.0%, 17.0% and 18.0% simultaneously had malaria, diarrhoea and acute respiratory infection (ARI), respectively, and 122 (87.8%) of those malnourished children had at least one or more of these three diseases.

Conclusion The nutritional status of children in Mogadishu IDP camps seems to be worsening if compared to the UNICEF survey of IDP camps in July 2004. On the other hand, the prevalence of malaria, ARI and diarrhoea seems to have improved in the current report.

Background

The ongoing conflict situation hampers access to the most-needy areas. A United Nations Children's Fund (UNICEF) survey conducted in Mogadishu internally displaced person (IDP) camps showed a prevalence of acute respiratory infection (ARI) (39.6%), diarrhoea (39.8%) and malaria (22.6%), with a malnutrition status about 13.8% (UNICEF survey, July 2004). A 2005 report by Médecins Sans Frontières found that 10% of newborn babies died after birth and 25% died before their 5th year.

A study was therefore carried out to determine whether the situation regarding ARI, diarrhoea, malaria and malnutrition had changed. The overall objective was to study the prevalence and determinants of malaria, diarrhoea and ARI in children less than 5 years in IDP camps in Mogadishu. Specific objectives were to evaluate the nutritional status in children in these displaced populations and the associations between the children's nutrition status and each of these diseases; to increase mother's awareness about the means to improve the nutritional status of their children and the importance of breast feeding; and to educate them about importance of hygienic measures, the use of oral dehydration solution

Conclusions and implications of the study

- Security in IDP camps in Mogadishu has been much improved, especially after the Islamic Court Union has come to control in Mogadishu city. Nevertheless, the economic situation of households in the IDP camps has remained unchanged. The decline of humanitarian organizations' activities has added to the economic problems.
- Humanitarian agencies must increase activities to improve health services in the IDP camps.
- Intensive health education activity should be set up in the camps, in order to improve personal hygiene and general environmental conditions.
- Households should be educated in proper waste disposal in their dwellings.
- Intensive education activities should be directed to mothers to promote exclusive breastfeeding practices; promote use of oral rehydration solutions for diarrhoea episodes; increase preventive measures for malaria (use of insecticides and bednets); and promote early health-seeking behaviour at the onset of respiratory symptoms.
- Intensive immunization, especially of children, should be provided to promote community defence mechanisms.

for diarrhoeal episodes, preventive measures for malaria (use of insecticide-treated bednets) and adequate health-seeking behaviour with onset of symptoms.

Materials and methods

A cross-sectional observational surveillance study with nested case–control phase was conducted in Mogadishu IDP camps. The target population was children 6–59 months of age, or 65–110 cm, living in IDP camps. The sampling technique was a multistage cluster sampling technique. It consisted first of random selection of districts and villages (camps) to be surveyed, then random selection of households and, finally, selection of one child in each household. The survey team was composed of four groups, with three interviewers in each group. All 12 interviewers were well trained and had extensive field experience. One team leader was responsible for record keeping and one for anthropometric measurements.

The interviewers used well-designed, structured questionnaires to gather the required information from the head of the household (mother) regarding the sociodemographic status of the selected household and to determine the risk factors for malaria, ARI and diarrhoea. Anthropometric measurements were recorded for each child.

Main study findings

Nine hundred (900) children were examined in Mogadishu IDP camps; 51% were boys. Global and severe acute malnutrition was 15.4% (95% confidence interval, CI: 19.3%–11.4%) and 3.3% (95% CI: 7.2%–1.0%), respectively, and 14.8% and 16.2% of boys and girls, respectively, were malnourished.

Moderate malnutrition (Z_scores < -2 and > -3) was observed more frequently in the 12–23 months and 24–35 months age groups (4.0% and 3.6%), respectively. While severe malnutrition (Z_scores < -3) was highest (1.6%) in the 24–35 months age group. This correlation between age and malnutrition was statistically significant ($P = 0.023$). Of these malnourished children, 8.0%, 17.0% and 18.0% simultaneously had malaria, diarrhoea and ARI, respectively, and 122 (87.8%) of those malnourished children had at least one or more of these three diseases.

The prevalence of diarrhoeal diseases was higher among children under 2 years of age (8.6% and 16.4% in the 6–11 and 12–23 months age groups, respectively). While ARI affected more children between 2 and 5 years of age (13.7%, 9.6% and 6.8% in 24–35, 36–47 and 48–59 months age groups, respectively). The relationship between the three diseases and malnutrition was highly significant ($P = 0.006$).

Conclusions and recommendations

The nutritional status of children in Mogadishu IDP camps seems to be worsening if compared to the UNICEF survey of IDP camps in July 2004, which showed global wasting rates of 13.8% (95% CI: 12.8%–19.6%) and a severe acute malnutrition rate of 3.2% (CI 2.2%–4.7%). On the other hand, the prevalence of malaria (22.6%), ARI (39.6%) and diarrhoea (35.8%) in the 2004 UNICEF survey seems to have improved in the current report.

Yemen

Leprosy

Integration of leprosy services into primary health-care services at district level in Yemen

- **Yemen**
  Nationwide
- **Study period**
  November 2006–July 2007
- **Small Grants Scheme**
  (SGS) 2006 No. 69

- **Principal Investigator**
  Yasin Al-Qubati
  Ministry of Public Health and Population
  Taiz, Yemen
  e-mail: nlep@y.net.ye

Abstract

A pilot study was conducted in Yemen to evaluate the effectiveness of integrating leprosy-control services into primary health care services at the district level. A total of 127 primary health-care workers (PHCWs) were selected from eight districts that are endemic with leprosy. Pre- and post-testing were carried out on the PHCWs to evaluate their knowledge, attitude and leprosy-diagnosis ability after 1 day of extensive training.

Results Following the educational seminars, the PHCWs demonstrated an increased overall knowledge about leprosy and its management. More than half (53%) of the PHCWs scored above 50% in the post-test, while only 3% scored above 50% in the pretest. There was also a 53% increase in the leprosy case detection in the same pre- and post-training period.

Conclusion The results showed a marked improvement in knowledge about leprosy after training and a moderate improvement in case detection of new cases of early leprosy by the trained PHCWs at the district and subdistrict level. In hypoendemic areas, leprosy control becomes difficult and the need for integration with PHCWs is essential. However, achievement will be lower than expectation, so monitoring, follow-up and supervision will be essential for the maintenance of integrated leprosy-control services.

Integrating leprosy-control services into primary health care services at the district level is the most effective way of addressing the residual problem of leprosy by ensuring early diagnosis and better accessibility of multidrug therapy (MDT) and thus providing a practical and cost-effective method for the final push against leprosy according to the NLEP new global strategy guidelines for 2006–2010.

Background

Leprosy is an important health-care problem in Yemen; according to the National Leprosy Eradication Programme (NLEP), 400–500 new cases are detected each year. In 1989, the overall prevalence of leprosy was 2 per 10 000, which is higher than the 1991 declared WHO target of 1 per 10 000. The Ministry of Health in Yemen, in cooperation with the German Leprosy and TB Relief Association, started the NLEP over the past decade and has made great progress, reflected by the decrease in the prevalence of leprosy to 0.2 per 10 000; however, the incidence of leprosy remains the same. Continuation of a vertical approach for leprosy control becomes costly and impractical. Integration of leprosy services into the available functioning primary health care services was an alternative solution.

A total of 127 primary health-care workers (PHCWs) were selected. Of these, nine were physicians and 118 were nurses representing eight districts in Yemen. All selected PHCWs from each district were invited for a 1-day comprehensive training workshop on leprosy and were asked to answer a well-designed pretest to assess their existing knowledge before training. Training was carried out according to NLEP guidelines for PHCWs, focusing on the diagnosis of the cardinal signs of leprosy, steps of the sensation test, classification, MDT, reaction recognition, treatment and registration. At the end of the day, the PHCWs were tested again and their test scores recorded.

Main study findings

The majority of the PHCWs had obtained information on leprosy mostly through previous official training courses conducted by the NLEP in centres in their governorates. Some had gained their knowledge through reading books or pamphlets distributed by the NLEP, or had seen leprosy

Conclusions and implications of the study

- Integration of leprosy-control activities into PHCSs is required for long-term sustainability of leprosy control in a cost-effective manner.
- Continued short-term focused training for PHCWs is essential for ensuring the effectiveness of integrating the leprosy-control services into PHCSs at the district level.
- Leprosy should be a real part of PHCSs in the periphery and in co-operation with dermatologists in the cities.

patients or suspected leprosy patients in their work. Over half (52%) of the PHCWs expressed a fear of stigma from leprosy.

In the pretest questionnaire, 82% were aware of the cause of leprosy and 48% knew its mode of transmission; however, only 27% could give one cardinal sign for the diagnosis of leprosy, only 21% could describe a part of the sensation test and only 25% could name a drug used in its treatment. In general, the pretest results were poor (97% scored a mark less than 50%). A marked increase in knowledge was demonstrated in the post-test, with 53% scoring a mark higher than 50% for the complete test, and 72% demonstrating knowledge of diagnosis of leprosy. The outcomes of the pre- and post-tests and the trained PHCW's attitudes towards leprosy patients varied slightly in the targeted areas.

In the period from November 2006 to July 2007, only 7% of the trained PHCWs were able to find and diagnose a total of 15 leprosy cases (47% multibacillary and 53% paucibacillary) and provide MDT to patients. The diagnosed cases were 53% male and 47% female (14 adults and 1 child), 87% had disability grade 0 and 13% had disability grade 2; another 4 cases were older, disabled leprosy cases who had already been treated in a leprosy clinic, while 18 other cases were ruled out by the leprosy focal point due to a wrong diagnosis.

The distribution of the 15 cases diagnosed by the PHCWs was as follows: 7 cases in Alzohra area; 7 cases in Doan; 1 case in Baitalfakih and no case diagnosed in Khanfar. The number of health facilities that found leprosy cases and provided MDT services was low (9 health facilities). Leprosy case detection in the same pre-and post-training period increased by 2.1 folds (from 7 to 15 cases) During the same period, the total number of cases detected by the leprosy focal points of the same areas was 21 compared to 35 cases in the previous year.

Conclusions and recommendations

The study showed an improvement in the PHCWs' knowledge of leprosy following training and also an increase in the diagnosis and case detection of leprosy cases after training. However, the number of cases detected by the PHCWs was lower compared with previous years, when active rapid skin surveys were implemented in the same areas the by leprosy mobile teams.

Malaria

Evaluation of the feasibility and acceptability of home management of malaria strategy adapted to Sudan's conditions using artemisinin-based combination therapies and rapid diagnostic tests

- **Sudan**
  Kordofan State
- **Study period**
  June–December 2007

- **Small Grants Scheme**
  (SGS) 2006 No. 47

- **Principal Investigator**
  Elfatih Mohamed Malik
  Communicable Diseases Control
  Federal Ministry of Health
  Khartoum, Sudan
  e.mail: fatihmmalik@hotmail.com

Abstract

The project aimed to test a model for home-based management of malaria (HMM) in Sudan. The model consisted of training malaria-control assistants in 43 villages in south-west Kordofan in the diagnosis of malaria using rapid diagnostic tests (RDTs) and treating malaria patients using artemisinin-based combination therapies (ACTs) recommended for malaria [coblister of artesunate and sulfadoxine–pyrimethamine (SP) and/or artesunate suppositories]. A community-based survey was carried out in 10 villages to assess the prevalence of malaria and the health-care-seeking behaviour of the community. Focus-group discussions were conducted as well as record surveys. Malaria control assistants (MCAs) were selected and trained and the situation was re-evaluated after the intervention.

Results All MCAs' registration and reports exceeded the minimum acceptable level of accuracy and 60% of them were excellent. Most (95%) of the MCAs adhered to the project design and attended scheduled meetings and submitted monthly reports.

In each village, a village-health committee was established from the available community leaders. These village health committees, together with the villagers, supported their MCA by providing a room to serve as a clinic. The system for ACTs and RDTs supply and distribution was effective since no MCA reported that stock had run out or complained of difficulties in replenishing stock.

The HMM project served a population of more than 23 000 residents. A total of 3745 patients were treated during the period June–December 2007. Of these, 17.6% (659 patients) were children under 5 years. During the same period, MCAs referred 35 (0.9%) cases to nearby hospitals with a diagnosis of a febrile condition other than malaria. MCAs reported 7 (0.2%) deaths in their respective villages, from various causes. MCAs also reported 7 (0.2%) cases of mild side-effects with ACT use. The study reported overall community satisfaction with the project.

Conclusion The study tested a pilot model for HMM implementation and reported its feasibility and positive impact on malaria control. It is recommended that the model is expanded all over the country and that other communicable diseases, such as diarrhoeal diseases and acute respiratory infections, are integrated into the model.

Background

Home-based malaria management (HMM) has recently become an official WHO strategy. In Ethiopia, malaria mortality was reduced by about 40% through training mothers to recognize malaria and give appropriate treatment at home. Different strategies have been used to try to implement HMM. The project aimed to implement and assess a model for HMM using artemisinin-based combination therapies (ACTs) recommended for malaria [coblister of artesunate and sulfadoxine–pyrimethamine (SP) and/ or artesunate suppositories and rapid diagnostic tests (RDT)] in Sudan.

Conclusions and implications of the study

- The study tested a pilot model for HMM implementation and reported its feasibility and positive impact on malaria control.
- It is recommended that this model is expanded all over the country and that other communicable diseases, such as diarrhoeal diseases and acute respiratory infections, are integrated into the model. Along with malaria, these diseases constitute the main killers for the under-5 years age group.
- All villagers were eager for the project to continue after the end of the pilot as it had helped to reduce the disease burden in their community. The system for ACTs and RDTs supply and distribution was effective and no MCA reported running out of stock or having difficulty replenishing stock.
- The introduction of this HHM model is especially important in communities that may be inaccessibility to health services during the rainy season.

Materials and methods

A quasi-experimental study was conducted in south-west Kordofan region (Um Adara area). There are 43 villages and a population of around 75 000, including nomads, in the area. This area was selected as there were sufficient data related to malaria/fever treatment-seeking behaviour. Malaria in the area is meso- to hyperendemic, with high and very long seasonal transmission (May–November). In general, the area is underdeveloped, the main occupations being farming and cattle breeding. There were three successive phases of the study.

Baseline phase

This phase consisted of a community household survey in 10 randomly selected villages in order to evaluate the health-seeking behaviour of the community and the prevalence of parasitaemia (symptomatic and preventive tools).

Focus-group discussions involving community leaders were held in the 10 selected villages to evaluate community preference for treatment and acceptability of HMM with a malaria-control assistant (MCA) providing care for malaria patients. Structured interviews with MCAs were conducted before and after the intervention to assess their views and any barriers regarding the intervention. Record-based surveys were also carried out at the health centres/facilities.

Implementation/intervention phase

In this phase, the MCA performed the RDTs and provided treatment for community members who sought care at home. A training protocol was developed for this purpose. The MCAs provided drugs for the target population closest to their residence area free of charge; however, there was a US$ 1 fee per person per consultation to motivate the MCAs and assist with the implementation of the scheme. Patients with negative RDT results were given antipyretics and referred to the nearest health centre if there was no clinical response within 48 h of starting treatment, or if the patient showed danger signs. Critically ill children were referred to a health centre immediately after receiving rectal artesunate.

MCA records and case reports used prepared registers. Supportive supervision and monitoring was conducted on a regular basis by the malaria control programme, using a check-list. The assistant pharmacist at the Um Adara health centre (the district health facility) distributed prepacked antimalarial drugs and RDTs to MCAs, to ensure a continuous supply of RDTs and drugs.

A sensitization and mobilization campaign was launched in the area at the beginning of the project. Communities were advocated to use HMM services.

Post-intervention phase

This phase consisted of post-intervention evaluation, using the same tools that were applied in the baseline phase.

Main study findings

The population survey, involving 200 households and their residents, revealed that the under-5 age group represented 40.1% of the population. The mean number of household members was 4.4. The female ratio was 61.9%. Malaria parasitological prevalence (pre-rainy season survey) was found to be 2.7% and *Plasmodium falciparum* was the only prevailing species. The number of malaria cases relative to house members in the previous season was between 40 and 100% and the number of malaria deaths within villages during the previous season ranged from 0 and 4, mostly children according to community leaders. The majority (98.5%) of the population sought treatment at public health facilities located between 2 km and 30 km from their home; 43.5% attended a facility over 10 km from their home.

Some villages had a community health worker within the village. Referred cases were transported during the rainy season by foot, donkey, carts, bicycles and cars; however, some villages were inaccessible. Community leaders listed the problems associated with malaria treatment as: accessibility to health services; high cost of drugs and difficulty finding drugs; treatment was on a clinical basis; treatment was sometimes unsatisfactory; and patients having to be referred elsewhere.

Mosquito nets were available in more than one third of households; of these more than 60% were insecticide-treated nets (ITNs) and more than 90% of these were long-lasting insecticide-treated nets (LLINs). However, despite this availability, only 2.9% had used bednets the previous night.

MCA performance

The 20 selected MCAs were male, with a mean age of 38.2 years. Their educational level varied. The main profession was farmer (50%) or health worker (40%), the remainder were merchants and employees. Forty-five per cent (45%) had previous experience of treating malaria.

Only one MCA did not adherent to treatment guidelines. Two MCAs had a problem with stock management and using and interpreting RDTs. Six MCAs (30%) treated patients based on clinical diagnosis, rather than relying on RDT results. All MCAs' registrations and reports exceeded the minimum acceptable level of accuracy and 60% of them were excellent. Most (95%) of the MCAs adhered to the project design and attended scheduled meetings and submitted monthly reports, while 65% of MCAs initiated educational and health-promotional activities, which were well supported in the community.

In each village, a health committee was established from the community leaders. Village health committees, together with the villagers, supported their MCA by providing a room to be used as a clinic. Most of village health committees were active in visiting their MCA in his clinic and/or house and discussing with him his work and any problems; 68.4% of committees had visited their MCA at least once every 2 months and only 21.1% had never visited their MCA. The majority (84.2%) of MCAs thought that the village health committees had a positive impact on their work.

The system for the supply and distribution of ACTs and RDTs was effective and no MCA ran out of stock or had difficulty replenishing their stock.

Quality of RDTs and drugs

Drugs and RDTs were satisfactory in their quality and performance, respectively. ACTs' quality was checked at the National Drugs Quality Control Laboratory. The performance of RDTs was measured against microscopy and showed a 97% and 100% sensitivity and specificity, respectively.

Treatment-seeking behaviour

Fever prevalence in the previous 2 weeks was 24% and 8.5% in the pre- and postintervention surveys, respectively. Of those who had fever, 83.3% sought treatment prior to the implementation of the HMM project; this increased to 100% after the implementation. Concerning severe malaria, 2 cases (1%) and 1 (0.5%) were observed within the 6 months before and after the availability of HMM services, respectively. Of these, 50% and 100%, respectively, were referred to hospital for treatment. There were 61 deaths (30.5%) in the season preceding the project, but only one (0.5%) after implementation of the project. Of these, 100% and 0.0% were under 5 years old and 4.9% and 0.0% were considered as malaria deaths for pre- and postintervention groups, respectively.

Patients treated by MCAs

The HMM project served a population of more than 23 000 residents and 3745 patients were treated during the period June–December, 2007. Of these, 17.6% (659 patients) were children under 5 years. During the same period, MCAs referred 35 (0.9%) cases to nearby hospitals, diagnosing them as having a febrile condition other than malaria. MCAs reported 7 (0.2%) deaths in their respective villages with variable causes of deaths. MCAs also reported 7 (0.2%) cases of mild side-effects coinciding with ACT use.

Satisfaction with the project

When HMM was discussed with village community leaders in focus groups, all participants said that they were aware that there was an MCA available in their village to diagnose and treat malaria cases and give advice for other conditions. They had discovered this through various channels. Those who made use of the HMM services acknowledged it was easy to access, nearby and cheap. They also mentioned that the selected MCAs were acceptable because of their honesty, the way they dealt with patients, had time for their patients as well as their own work, and because of their knowledge and ability.

Conclusions and recommendations

The model of implementation of HMM in Sudan was promising. The use of RDTs in such condition is fundamental since it helps to support diagnosis and also trust in MCAs. Although the project needs some adaptation, its general feasibility, acceptability and effectiveness were reported.

Malaria

Adherence of the private sector to the national malaria control programme guidelines in diagnosis, treatment and reporting of malaria patients in Afghanistan

- **Afghanistan**
  Malaria endemic provinces
- **Study period**
  August 2005–2006
- **Small Grants Scheme**
  (SGS) 2005 No. 60

- **Principal Investigator**
  Khalilahmad Kohestani
  Ministry of Public Health
  Kabul, Afghanistan
  e-mail: Khalil_impd@yahoo.com

Abstract

A study was conducted on the private-sector adherence to National Malaria and Leishmaniasis Control Programme (NMLCP) guidelines in diagnosis, treatment and reporting of malaria cases in 15 provinces in Afghanistan (14 with high-risk of malaria and one epidemic-prone province). A list of private-sector facilities was prepared for each province and 10% of the facilities randomly selected. A medical doctor and a laboratory technician from each facility were invited to participate in the study. A total of 189 health workers (117 medical doctors and 72 laboratory technicians) consented to participate in the study. They were invited to a workshop where they were given a self-administered questionnaire to evaluate their baseline knowledge about malaria in their province and to collect information on their referral practices, reporting practices, and opinions on involvement with national control efforts. They were then given an orientation session to improve their knowledge and increase their adherence to guidelines.

Results There was suboptimal knowledge regarding NMLCP guidelines in diagnosis, treatment and reporting of malaria cases in both groups during the intervention. However, the study also indicated great interest by private-service providers to participate in the NMLCP.

Conclusion The study highlighted the need to develop a strategy of collaboration between the public and private sector (public–private partnership), where the roles and responsibilities of the private sector are well defined.

Introduction

Afghanistan has a national policy framework for malaria control, the National Malaria Strategic Plan (NMSP), which is administered and overseen by the National Malaria and Leishmaniasis Control Programme (NMLCP) with support from a range of partners. The role played by the private sector in malaria control is of concern to the NMLCP. This role is seen as vital to the success of the disease-control strategy, given the high use of the private sector and the gaps in the developing public sector. However, relatively little is known about the current practice and role of the private sector.

The NMSP is calling for the private sector to actively participate in national malaria-control efforts. The first stage of such inclusion is to evaluate this sector's current practices and procedures in diagnosis, treatment and disease reporting, with the eventual aim of developing and implementing an accreditation scheme for private-sector practitioners. This will provide guidelines on "best practice", which will be a minimum standard of care available through the private sector. Practitioners would undertake training and assessment before being certified as "malaria specialists". The scheme would also be coupled to a public-awareness campaign advising the public to use private-sector malaria specialist facilities.

The objective of the study was to evaluate the extent of adherence of private health-care providers to NMLCP guidelines for diagnosis and treatment of malaria patients. It

Conclusions and implications of the study

- To improve the standard and level of involvement of private-sector practitioners in Afghanistan, a formal training and accreditation scheme needs to be designed and conducted as a pilot intervention. A comprehensive and concise curriculum needs to be developed, in collaboration with private-sector representatives. It should include basic knowledge of malaria and its control; diagnosis (including rapid diagnostic tests) and treatment according to national guidelines; health education; and reporting and disease surveillance.
- This scheme could be supervised by the NMLCP and its partners and conducted through malaria reference centres. After training and accreditation, practitioners would have a certificate. This training should be accompanied by a public-awareness campaign. Outcomes would be measured according to specific objective indicators.
- A system of service quality checking and retraining should be conducted.
- A quality-assurance scheme for antimalarial drugs should be implemented to ensure treatment uniformity and the possibility of a purchasing scheme should be considered.
- A case-reporting scheme should be piloted in the private sector, overseen by local health authorities and the NMLCP.

also sought to assess the extent of collaboration of the private health-care providers in reporting and referring malaria cases, where necessary, to the NMLCP.

Materials and methods

The study was conducted in 15 provinces in Afghanistan. These areas were chosen on the basis of being malaria endemic, with the exception of Bamyan, which was chosen as an epidemic-prone province. Other than Bamyan, the remaining provinces are classified as having high risk for malaria, based on surveillance data.

Participating private-sector units were selected from a list of facilities provided by the provincial Ministry of Public Health (MoPH). The sample was a convenience sample that aimed to include 10% of the clinics listed in each province. At each facility, the clinic doctor was asked to participate in the survey. Technicians randomly selected from a MoPH list were also asked to participate. A total of 189 health workers (117 medical doctors and 72 laboratory technicians) consented to participate in the study.

The health workers were invited to a workshop where they were given a self-administered questionnaire to evaluate baseline knowledge about malaria in their province (transmission season, case load, etc.) and to collect information on their referral practices, reporting practices, and opinions on their involvement with national control efforts. Data were also collected on the practice history and qualifications of participants. They were then given an orientation session to improve their knowledge and increase

Main study findings

Private practitioners

One hundred and seventeen (117) doctors agreed to participate in the study and be interviewed. Seven (6%) interviewees were female and 110 (94%) male. The age range was from 25 to 71 years, with a mean age of 39.7 years (standard deviation, SD 8.4); 22 (19%) had worked for less than 5 years in their profession and 94 (91%) for over 5 years. Of the interviewees, 98 (83.8%) had received official permission for private practice from the central MoPH, while 19 (16.2%) had received permission from the provincial MoPH; 95 (81.2%) held an official job in addition to their private-practice activities, while 22 (18.2%) received their sole income from their private practice. Of the 95 with other employment, 80 (84.2%) worked for the government and 15 (15.8%) worked for nongovernmental organizations (NGOs). The number of days per week that private-service providers worked in their clinic varied from 4 to 7 days (mean 6.3 days, SD 0.6). Regarding motivation, 40 (34.2%) regarded their private practice as a service to the people, 17 (14.5%) stated economic reasons for private practice and 60 (51.3%) claimed both factors as motivation.

Malaria-specific data

Of 116 responders, 60 (51.7%) had attended one or more malaria refresher courses, 113 (97.4%) responders saw between 1 and 1200 malaria suspects per month (mean 126, SD 189.2, median 60) and 111 (95.7%) reported to have seen between 0 to 300 malaria cases in the previous month (mean 47.9, SD 67.9, median 17).

Of the 117 interviewees, 78 (67.8%) used blood examinations to diagnose malaria, 5 (4.3%) diagnosed malaria clinically and 32 (27.8%) used both methods, and 2 referred the cases for diagnosis. For confirmation, 17 (14.5%) sent patients to nearby public-sector health facilities, 91 (77.8%) used private laboratories and 9 (7.7%) used both; 111 (94.9%) said their nearby health facility had laboratory facilities capable of performing malaria confirmatory tests.

Regarding treatment, 115 of the interviewees (98.3%) stated that they had treated malaria cases in their clinic. Of these, 113 answered the question about the treatment regimen used; 63 (55.8%) claimed to follow NMLCP's national protocol and 50 (44.2%) used other treatment regimens. Of the 115 who treated malaria, 83 (72.2%) claimed to have a follow-up system for *Plasmodium falciparum* cases. Only 32 of those treating malarial cases (27.8%) reported these cases to the MoPH, with 83 (72.2%) not reporting them.

Of 117 responders, only 36 (30.8%) had received at least one supervisory visit from a MoPH representative in the past, while the remaining 81 (60.2%) had never received any such visits. A statistically significant relationship was demonstrated between private-service providers receiving supervisory visits from the MoPH and their adherence to national treatment guidelines. A total of 25 of the 34 (69.5%) practitioners who had received supervisory visits claimed to use the national protocol.

Regarding restrictions to the use of antimalarial drugs, 36 of the 117 interviewees (30.8%) thought that antimalarial drugs should only be available in the government/ public sector, whereas 81 (69.2%) thought that these drugs should be available in both public and private sectors.

Regarding surveillance, 95 of 117 responders (81.2%) believed they could play a positive role in supporting the country's malaria surveillance system; of these, 79 (83.2%) thought they could participate in data reporting, 15 (15.8%) offered to provide outbreak information, while 1 (1.1%) stated other roles.

Of the 117 interviewees, 109 (93.2%) were willing/able to participate in malaria control activities of the NMLCP. However, when asked later if they would agree to co-operate with the NMLCP for malaria-control activities in the future, 114 (98.3%) said that they would; 78 of these (68.4%) would expect to receive support for their participation, whereas 36 (31.6%) would not expected support. Of the 78 who expected support, 35 (44.9%) expected both financial and technical support, 13 (16.7%) expected financial support only and 30 (38.5%) expected only technical support.

To assess general knowledge about malaria, interviewees were asked about malaria peak seasons in their area, when they would advise slide examinations for malaria, and about referral of malaria patients to hospital. Of 103 responders to the question on *Plasmodium vivax* peak season, 11 (10.7%) correctly identified it as summer; 90 (87.4%) placed it in autumn, which is partially correct since the malaria season stretches from June to November and there are many cases still seen in autumn. Two responders wrongly identified winter as the peak season for *Plasmodium vivax* transmission.

Of 112 responders to the question on *Plasmodium falciparum* peak season, only 5 (4.5%) correctly identified autumn as its peak season; 104 (92.9%) identified summer as the peak season and 3 (2.7%) even thought it would be spring.

Regarding febrile patients, 108 of the 117 interviewees (92.3%) advised slide examinations for all febrile patients, while the remaining 9 (7.7%) advised slide examinations for all febrile patients and referral of malaria suspects. A total of 84 of the 117 (71.8%) would refer some malaria cases to hospitals; of these, 27 (23.1%) would refer comatose patients, 36 (42.9%) seriously ill patients, 12 (14.3%) treatment failures, 8 (9.5%) febrile cases and 1 (1.2%) stated other reasons.

Laboratory technicians

Seventy-two (72) laboratory technicians were interviewed; their mean age was 37 years, 90% were male, 36% held a baccalaureate degree (i.e. finished high school), 47% held a technologist certificate/diploma, 6% were MDs and 11% stated other education levels. Most (72%) had worked for more than 5 years.

Only 13% worked without official permission and 56 (78%) held an official job in addition to their private practice. Of these 56, 80% worked for the government and 20% for NGOs. When asked their reasons for operating a private practice, 50% stated both economical reasons and the desire to provide a service for the people, 28% stated economic reasons alone, and 22% stated only a desire to provide a service for the people.

Technicians saw an average of 200 slides per month (range 8–1500), with a slide positivity rate (SPR) of 10–30% reported by the majority of respondents (80%). This SPR directly corresponded with previous experience. Most (> 90%) work for 6 or 7 days per week.

A total of 80% believed malaria to be a serious public-health problem, and 97% reported a willingness to be involved in malaria control. The majority (94%) would like to have cross-checking (quality assurance) provided for them, although only 50% kept the slides that they had used for diagnosis. Half (50%) reported having had a supervisory visit from MoPH staff. All participants said they would take part in malaria surveillance and 58% kept a malaria register.

Regarding diagnosis technique, only 58% conducted both thick and thin smears (the gold standard), 35% performed only thick smears and 7% only thin smears needed to identify the parasite species.

A total of 40% had attended more than two malaria microscopy refresher courses, 33% had attended one or two courses, but 27% had not attended any course. There appeared to be no correlation between having an "official job" and training, as 75% of those with and those without official jobs had attended training. Thus, where available, training courses were well attended by private sector practitioners.

Conclusions and recommendations

The study reported suboptimal adherence of the private sector to national guidelines for case management of malaria and in reporting practices to the NMLCP. However, the study also showed that private practitioners were willing to be included in NMLCP disease-control efforts, and that they were receptive to training schemes organized by the programme.

Malaria

Confirmation of malaria using rapid diagnostic tests: appraisal for stability, accuracy and acceptance by health providers and community in eastern Sudan

- **Sudan**
  Kassala State
- **Study period**
  November 2005–April 2006
- **Small Grants Scheme**
  (SGS) 2005 No. 140

- **Principal Investigator**
  Osama M.E. Seidahmed
  National Malaria and Leishmania Control Programme
  Federal Ministry of Health
  Khartoum, Sudan
  e-mail: malarsud@hotmail.com

Abstract

The study aimed to evaluate the diagnostic performance of two rapid diagnostic tests (RDTs) for the diagnosis of malaria: Core Malaria Pf [histidine-rich protein 2, (HRP2)-based] and OptiMAL-IT [parasite lactate dehydrogenase (pLDH)-based]. It also aimed to evaluate their stability and end-user practice under field conditions. The two RDT kits were kept under field conditions within cupboards at six selected health dispensaries. A total of 734 symptomatic patients attending six peripheral health dispensaries at Halfa El Gedida in Sudan were enrolled during the period November 2005–April 2006 and tested using both RDTs. For each patient, examination of blood smears was carried out blinded to the patient record. The study also evaluated end-user errors during the preparation of the tests and interpretation of the results. In addition, community acceptance was appraised by interviewing a subsample of patients who had been tested by the RDTs.

Results Of the 734 patients, 79 (10.8%) were confirmed malaria cases. For the Core Malaria Pf (Core Diagnostics, UK) and OptiMAL-IT (DiaMed AG, Switzerland) tests, sensitivity values were 96% and 50%, and specificity values were 97% and 98%, respectively. The Core Malaria Pf test did not detect two of 47 *Plasmodium falciparum* infections, and it generated false-positive results for nine patients. The OptiMAL-IT test failed to detect 20 of 30 *P. falciparum* infections, and one of two infections of *P. vivax*, and it generated seven false-positive results.

Excessive temperatures above 30 °C were documented in all storage cupboards throughout the study period. While the storage time in the field affected the accuracy of both OptiMAL-IT and Core Malaria Pf, field temperature only affected stability of OptiMAL-IT and had no effect on the latter.

By using the manufacturer's instructions, preparation and interpretation of the dipstick format, OptiMAL-IT was considerably subject to end-user error compared with the cassette format of Core Malaria Pf. Two types of errors were reported: the generic-based errors that were common to both tests and not linked to the design of the test; and specific-based errors that are linked to the format, type and manufacturer's instructions of the tests. Furthermore, patients accepted consequent treatment based on RDTs and identified benefits of RDT diagnosis in this remote area.

Conclusion In view of the low prevalence of falciparum malaria at this peripheral health setting and the rarity of vivax malaria occurring without coinfection with the former, RDTs of HRP2-type that detect only *P. falciparum* are generally recommended to the malaria-control programme, particularly on grounds of lack of microscopy and reasonable cost.

The study appraised the use of a HRP2-brand of RDTs in tropical and remote areas. Logistical arrangements such as improving transport and storage conditions (e.g. developing cool chains) and shortening storage periods at the periphery health system (particularly during summer season) should be considered in order to avoid damage of RDTs.

Improving the practice on RDTs may require not only the construction of job aids but also appropriate training for end-users and, more significantly, minimizing human error by manufacturing tests with very simple instructions.

Conclusions and implications of the study

- The diagnostic performance of the Core Malaria Pf RDT (HRP2-based) was significantly higher than the OptiMAL-IT RDT (pLDH-based). It was more accurate and stable under field conditions.
- Storage and transport conditions can greatly affect the diagnostic performance of RDTs. Logistical arrangements, such as improving transport and storage conditions (e.g. developing cold chains) and shortening storage periods at the periphery health system (particularly during summer season) should be considered in order to avoid damage of RDTs.
- Several end-user errors were reported in the study. These can be minimized by appropriate training, regular supervision, and provision of job aids. Manufacturing tests with simpler instructions could also reduce these types of human errors.

Background

Rapid diagnostic tests (RDTs) have recently been introduced for situations where symptom-based diagnosis is the predominant methodology of managing suspected malaria cases. These RDTs are classified according to their antigen targets into three types. The first type is the histidine-rich protein 2 (HRP-2) based RDT, which involves a water-soluble protein produced by asexual young gametocyte stages of *Plasmodium falciparum*. The second type of RDT employs parasite lactate dehydrogenase (pLDH); this enzyme is produced by all blood-stage parasites and has isomers for each *Plasmodium* spp. The third type of RDT, which is less available commercially, employs an enzyme called plasmodium aldolase, which is produced by the four species of *Plasmodium*.

The sensitivity and specificity of each of these tests have been assessed in a range of clinical situations and there is a constant need to evaluate the effectiveness of RDTs at peripheral health settings, where these tests are to be used. This study was conducted at peripheral health dispensaries in rural areas of Halfa El Gedida, Sudan where malaria infection is endemic. These peripheral health dispensaries form the primary health-care centres at these sites and lack microscopy services to confirm malaria infection. The objective of this study was to determine effectiveness of two brands of RDTs: Core Malaria Pf (Core Diagnostics, UK) and OptiMAL-IT (Diamed AG, Switzerland) in suspected malaria patients presenting to peripheral health dispensaries. Core Malaria Pf is a HRP2-based type of RDT while OptiMAL-IT is a pLDH-type. Microscopy was used as a reference standard for comparisons of effectiveness. The study also aimed to evaluate their stability and end-user practice under field conditions.

Materials and methods

The study was carried out in Halfa El Gadida (15. 19 N; 35.36 E), Kassala state, east Sudan. Six health dispensaries, one per village, were selected. Criteria of the selection were: services of the dispensary were the sole unit of the periphery health system at these villages and also no microscopy service was available the dispensary.

Health providers (primary health workers, PHW), one per study site, were recruited to perform the RDTs. The PHWs were provided with appropriate training on the performance of Core Malaria Pf and OptiMAL-IT, according to manufacturer's instructions. A total of 734 patients who had fever, or had history of fever during the previous week, and who were clinically diagnosed by the health provider as symptomatic cases of uncomplicated malaria were enrolled in the study and tested by both RDTs.

For each patient, 100 thick-blood-smear fields were examined systemically for the presence of malaria parasites according to WHO criteria; blood smears were declared as negative after examination of 100 thick blood smears without detecting any malaria parasite. Thin blood smears were used for the identification of malaria species where appropriate. Examination of blood smears was carried out blinded to the patient record. Two senior microscopists examined the blood smears and all positive slides and a random selection of 10% of the negative slides were further checked by an expert technician.

RDT kits were kept under field conditions within a cupboard at each one of the selected dispensaries during the period November 2005–April 2006. In order to monitor storage conditions, a hygro thermometer (Sisedo hygrotherm™) was inserted inside each storage cupboard. Daily measurements of temperature and relative humidity inside the cupboards were made at 13:00 hours.

End-user practice of RDTs was monitored by the researchers during the monthly surveys using a checklist. The checklist was designed by the research team to obtain comparative and quantitative data on the preparation and interpretation of RDT by the PHWs. The researchers observed the practice of a total of 733 RDT devices.

Finally, a group discussion was conducted with end-users and researchers at the end of the study, to collect qualitative data on difficulties regarding the instructions of the two types of RDTs.

At the end of the study, 30 patients or their guardians who had previously been diagnosed for malaria using RDTs, were randomly selected from each study site and interviewed using a pretested questionnaire on their acceptance of their RDT results and their consequent treatment.

Main study findings

Of 734 enrolled patients, 398 (54.3%) were females and 107 (14.7%) were less than 5 years of age. Clinical examination by the PHWs revealed the immediate presence of fever in 236 (39.1%) patients and/or history of fever during the previous week in 538 (73.4%) patients. A total of 79 patients (prevalence = 10.8%) were found positive under microscopy, of which 76 (10.4%) and 2 (0.2%) specimens were diagnosed by thin blood smears as *P. falciparum* and *P. vivax*, respectively.

Performance of RDTs

A total of 71 positive malaria cases (average prevalence = 9.7%) were obtained for both types of RDTs, of which 17 cases were diagnosed by OptiMAL-IT (prevalence = 7.67%; 95% confidence interval, CI: 7.7%–7.7%), and 54 cases were detected by Core Malaria Pf (prevalence = 12.74%; 95% CI: 12.7%–12.7%). While 69 patients were diagnosed as having P. falciparum infection, only two cases of non-falciparum malaria were diagnosed using OptiMAL-IT, one of which was confirmed later as *P. vivax*. In addition, 78 results of OptiMAL-IT were rejected as invalid.

The diagnostic performance of Core Malaria Pf RDT was significantly higher than the OptiMAL-IT RDT; sensitivity, specificity, positive and negative predictive values of Core Malaria Pf RDT were 96%, 97%, 83% and 99% versus 50%, 98%, 65% and 96%, respectively.

Regarding stability, in contrast to Core Malaria Pf, where no invalid devices were obtained, 78 invalid OptiMAL-IT devices were obtained. The number of unstable OptiMAL-IT devices was significantly correlated with both the mean storage temperature of cupboards and the storage months in the field, 33 unstable devices of OptiMAL-IT were obtained when storage temperature exceeded 37 °C on 6 April.

Regarding accuracy, 358 (97%) devices of Core Malaria Pf were found to be accurate, compared with 270 (74%) of OptiMAL-IT devices. A significant inverse correlation between the proportion of accurate devices of OptiMAL-IT and field-temperature was obtained.

Errors with generic measurements were observed. End-users had not regarded the written instructions while using 697 (95.7%) devices, only using instructions in 31 sessions. Difficulties were observed during blood collection from the patients and during blood transfer to strips during 55 (7.5%) and 32 (4.4%) sessions, respectively. Stopwatches had been provided to the six health dispensaries during the first survey and were regularly used by the end-users to measure timing of the RDTs. Although many 694 RDT devices (96.3%) were used at night, the light was adequate in the health dispensaries to read the results.

Errors with specific measurements were also observed, for example failure by the end-user to blot a suitable blood volume in the sample well or their incorrect positioning of devices.

Regarding adherence to the manufacturer's instructions, the end-users conducted all the test steps either for Core Malaria Pf (eight steps) or OptiMAL-IT (nine steps). However, other errors were observed, such as not following the order of the steps or blotting the buffer in a wrong place, spending longer or shorter time in testing, or wrongly interpreting results.

Group discussion and community acceptance

The group discussion showed a general agreement among end-users that the cassette Core Malaria Pf was easy to use compared with the dipstick OptiMAL-IT.

Regarding community acceptance of diagnosis by RDT, out of 177 patients (total from all sites) interviewed on their preference for malaria diagnosis, 101 said that diagnosis was a desirable procedure regardless of the method (microscopy or RDT). A total of 155 respondents said they would trust the use of RDTs in the future for malaria illness. Other reasons given by respondents for future reliance on RDTs included their accessibility in home situations, particularly in emergencies (17.3%) and avoiding the misuse of antimalarials (16.5%).

Conclusions and recommendations

In view of the low prevalence of falciparum malaria at these peripheral health settings and the rarity of vivax malaria occurring without coinfection with the former, RDTs of HRP2-type that detect only *P. falciparum* are generally recommended to the malaria-control programme, particularly on grounds of lack of microscopy and affordable cost.

Several end-user errors were reported by this study. Improving practice on RDTs may require not only the construction of job aids but also conduction of appropriate training for end-users, and more significantly minimizing human interference through manufacturing tests with very simple instructions.

Malaria

Estimation of malaria burden in Hadramout mesoendemic coastal districts, Yemen

- **Yemen**
  Hadramout Governate
- **Study period**
  December 2005–2006

- **Small Grants Scheme**
  (SGS) 2005 No. 184

- **Principal Investigator**
  Yahia Ahmed Raja'a
  Faculty of Medicine and Health Sciences
  Sana'a University
  Sana'a, Yemen
  e-mail: yahiarajaa@yahoo.com

Abstract

A study was carried out to estimate malaria burden in Hadramout Governorate and to evaluate the health-care-seeking behaviour of the community and the community's use of protective measures. The study design was a survey follow-up. The cross-sectional phase involved a parasitological survey of a randomly selected representative sample of the target population of Hadramout coastal districts, and took place during the first transmission season in the calendar year of the study (December 2005); 916 household members in 226 households were interviewed using a structured and pretested questionnaire. This phase was succeeded by a follow-up phase, wherein the whole village population was informed about the study and asked to report to the nearby health facility in case of febrile illness during the following calendar year.

Results In the household cross-sectional survey, the prevalence of asymptomatic parasitaemia was 26.0%. Only 2 houses out of 226 (0.9%) had screens on the windows and doors. Regular indoor residual spraying was reported in 110 houses out of 226 (48.7%). A total of 54 households out of 226 had mosquito nets (23.9%), 43 of these had treated nets and 41 had long-lasting treated nets. In total, 26.7% of the houses were reported to be suitable for mosquito breeding. The distance between homes and permanent mosquito-breading sites ranged from 0 to 1 km, with a median of 0.5 km. The total number of malaria cases recorded in the health facilities of the districts studied during the period from 1 January to 31 December 2006 was 171 out of a population of 80 975, giving an incidence rate of 211 per 100 000 population. The symptomatic/asymptomatic ratio was 1:123.

Conclusion The prevalence rate of asymptomatic malaria in the cross-sectional survey was 26%. Total recorded cases over the year following the cross-sectional survey were very low (171 cases), suggesting a symptomatic/asymptomatic ratio of 1:123. This wide gap could be attributed to the health-seeking behaviour of the population and their perception of febrile illness.

Background

In Yemen, malaria is the most common health problem. Rates obtained from field studies are substantially higher than rates based on health records; e.g. a field study carried out in Hajr Valley in Hadramout Governorate revealed a parasite rate of 13% and a spleen rate of 11% in children aged 6–11 years, whereas surveillance reports in the same governorate gave lower rates, e.g. 1.2% of all febrile cases were clinically diagnosed as malaria. Predicting incidence in the community from suitable indicators (e.g. notified cases or recorded febrile illnesses) would serve as an invaluable tool for the National Malaria Control Programme to prioritize and control the disease. The aim of the study was to estimate

Conclusions and implications of the study

- The study reported a low and inadequate use of malaria-protective measures. A health-education campaign, to improve health-seeking behaviour in the community and promote the use of protective measures, is highly recommended.
- Around half (50.2%) of the houses in the study area were built of mud and grass, thus provided a suitable breeding environment for the vector. More than one quarter (26.7%) of households were in debt by the end of the month. The highest incidence of malaria was in May, which could either be a reflection of the climate or be an epidemic, as suggested by the malaria-control project in the area. Climatic conditions, socioeconomic status and environmental factors all enhance malaria transmission.
- The health authority's input in the control of the disease was quite good, as 48.7% of households reported that their houses had regular indoor residual spraying.
- Over 80% of all households claimed to seek health care at public or private health facilities. However, their concept of illness may not have included febrile illness, as we found that almost all cases of fever had not been attributed to malaria.
- Almost half (48%) of the population in the studied districts were more than half an hour from their nearest health facility.
- The median cost of antimalarial drugs was US$ 5 for one episode, a sum of money greater than the daily wage of a low-hierarchy governmental worker (around US$ 3.5) and 35% of respondents could not afford to pay for such treatment.

malaria burden in Hadramout Governorate and to evaluate the health-care-seeking behaviour of the community and their use of protective measures.

Materials and methods

The study design was a survey follow-up. The cross-sectional phase involved a parasitological survey of a randomly selected representative sample of the target population of Hadramout coastal districts, which took place during the first transmission season in the calendar year of the study (December 2005). Selected subjects were interviewed using a structured and pretested questionnaire that included questions regarding sociodemographic variables; presence of breeding sites (indoor and outdoor); health-care-seeking behaviour; health-care accessibility; duration of illness; and use of protective measures.

This phase was succeeded by a follow-up phase, whereby the whole village population was informed about the study and asked to report to a nearby health facility in case of febrile illness occurring during the following calendar year. Households were randomly selected within each village and any febrile case occurring in these households during the study period (one calendar year) were examined clinically and subjected to blood examination for the malaria parasite. In this phase, data were also collected regarding the number of notified cases from each studied cluster (district/village). These data were obtained from the monthly medical records of the health facilities within each cluster during the phase duration.

Main study findings

In the household cross-sectional survey in the studied coastal districts of Hadramout, prevalence of asymptomatic parasitaemia was 26.0%. Asymptomatic parasitaemia was highest in the Al-Mukalla suburb. A total of 21.5% of the households had no children under 5 years.

Regarding construction of houses, 41.3% were constructed of stone but around half were built of mud and grass, i.e. materials suitable for mosquito survival. In addition, 26.7% were reported to be suitable for mosquito breeding. The distance between houses and permanent mosquito-breading sites ranged from 0 to 1 km, with a median of 0.5 km. Only 0.9% of houses had screens on windows and doors. Regular indoor residual spraying was reported in 48.7% of houses. A total of 24% had mosquito nets; of those individuals who had mosquito nets, 77.8% reported that these nets were treated. Of those who had a personal mosquito net, 92.6% had slept under the net the previous night. The majority of households (82.5%) believed that the nets were useful for malaria prevention.

Those who perceived their socioeconomic status as high (12.9%) reported that they had some monthly savings, 60.4% of the households reported that their income was equal to their expenses, while 26.7% said they had debts by the end of the month. Regarding educational level of the household principal, 55.7% reported a basic educational level, 42% had not had any formal education and 2.3% had attained university level or above.

Most of the respondents sought treatment at public health facilities (77%), 3.3% at private practitioners, 6.7% at traditional healers, while 13.3% reported self-treatment. The distance to their nearest health facility ranged from less than 1 km to as much as 100 km, with a median of 1 km; however, 86% reported a distant of 7 km or less. The time to reach the nearest health facility was less than half an hour in 51.8% of cases, but 21.6% took more than an hour to reached their nearest health facility. Almost half of the respondents (46.9%) reached their health facility on foot.

Antimalarial drugs were present in 1.3% of the surveyed houses. The cost of antimalarial drugs for one episode ranged between US$ 2.5 and US$ 100, with a median of US$ 5. A total of 65% said that they could afford to pay for treatment, while 35% said they could not afford to pay. A total of 8.7% of household members had been treated for malaria during the previous 2 weeks and 5.9% reported that a household member currently had fever. Of those, 47.2% had been febrile for less than 24 hours. The majority of those with fever (79.4%) had sought treatment, almost half of these (48.3%) within 24 hours. A total of 44.8% of those with fever were receiving treatment at the time of the interview.

Of the respondents with a household member with a febrile illness, all but one said that the cause of the fever was not malaria. In the malaria case, diagnosis had been carried out by blood examination in a health facility in Arreadeh. None of the febrile cases reported a recent history of travelling to a highly endemic area.

The total number of malaria cases recorded in the health facilities of the studied districts during the period from 1 January to 31 December 2006 was 171, out of a population of 80 975, giving an incidence rate of 211 per 100 000 population. The symptomatic/asymptomatic ratio was 1:123. The highest incidence of malaria was found in May.

Conclusions and recommendations

The prevalence rate of asymptomatic malaria found in the cross-sectional survey was 26%; the highest rate was found in the Al-Mukalla suburb. Recorded cases in the year following the cross-sectional survey were very low (171 cases). This suggests a symptomatic/asymptomatic ratio of 1:123. This wide gap could be attributed to the health-seeking behaviour

Estimating malaria burden in hypo–mesoendemic and hyperendemic areas in Sudan

- **Sudan**
  Nationwide
- **Study period**
  December 2005–February 2006

- **Small Grants Scheme**
  (SGS) 2005 No. 141 and (SGS) 2005 No. 154

- **Principal Investigator**
  Hatim Sid Ahmed Mustafa and Hmooda Toto
  National Malaria and Leishmania Control Programme
  Wad Madani, Gezira State
  State Ministry of Health, Sudan
  e-mail: malarsud@hotmail.com

Abstract

The study aim was to estimate the current malaria burden in different epidemiological settings in order to build a sensitive model for future estimation of malaria in Sudan. The study was carried out in two hypo–mesoendemic areas (Elhosh and Elmatama) and two hyperendemic areas (Malakal and Elrank). The study design included two phases. The initial, cross-sectional phase was conducted in randomly selected households in the two areas and consisted of a parasitological survey and interviews using a questionnaire. Individuals living in households randomly selected for the cross-sectional phase were encouraged to report to health facilities in the catchment area in case of any febrile illness during the study period. In the second, follow-up phase, the records from the health facilities that registered the cases within the catchment area were used by the study team on a monthly basis.

Results The prevalence of parasitaemia, fever and confirmed malaria at the time of the survey was 3.3%, 21.6% and 13.0%, respectively, in the Malakal area and 0.95%, 16.2% and 5.0%, respectively, in the Elrank area. The prevalence of parasitaemia, fever and confirmed malaria at the time of the survey was 1.9%, 13.3% and 3.8%, respectively, in the Elhosh area and 0.1%, 6.0% and 2.8%, respectively, in the Elmatama area.

The incidence of malaria episodes during the follow-up period was estimated to be 8.5 (980/125 901) and 178.6 (3526/47 384) per 1000 population in the Malakal (11 months) and Elrank (5 months) areas, respectively. The incidence of malaria episodes during the follow-up period was estimated to be 23.7 (2970/150 430) and 10.3 (482/80 000) per 1000 population in the Elhosh (10 months) and Elmatama (7 months) areas, respectively.

Using the prediction equation, the relationship between malaria incidence and the product of the symptomatic and asymptomatic ratio (S/AS) and prevalence was studied in the different areas and plotted.

Conclusion Using the prediction equation will allow estimations of incidence of malaria episodes in the future, based on the results of prevalence surveys in hypo-mesoendemic and hyperendemic areas.

Background

In Sudan, there are 7.5 million estimated malarial cases and 35 000 deaths from malaria every year. These estimations are based on previous Federal Ministry of Health annual statistical reports. The main limitations of these estimations include: low coverage (in place and time) of the ongoing health information system; many malaria cases are self-treated at home; suboptimal data quality; and misdiagnosis of any febrile illness as malaria. Therefore, there is a need for developing an estimation model that considers these limitations. This study aimed to estimate the current malaria burden in different epidemiological settings, in order to build a sensitive model for future estimation of malaria in Sudan.

Materials and methods

The study was carried out in two hypo-mesoendemic areas and two hyperendemic areas. The two areas representing the hyperendemic strata in Sudan were the Malakal and Elrank areas in Upper Nile State (southern Sudan). The two areas representing the hypo–mesoendemic strata in Sudan were the Elmatama and Elhosh areas in River Nile (desert-fringe along the River Nile) and Gezira (irrigated) States, respectively. The rainy season begins in July and continues to September.

The cross-sectional/follow-up study design had two phases. The cross-sectional phase was conducted in January

Conclusions and implications of the study

- In the absence of a strong health information system in developing countries, different epidemiological methods should be evaluated in order to determine the disease burden.
- The study has developed a new method for estimating malaria burden in different epidemiological settings, based on mathematical modelling and biological information. Testing its validity in future studies is recommended.

2006, just after the malaria season, in both hyperendemic areas (Malakal and Elrank), in December 2005 (at the end of the season) in the Elhosh area and in February 2006 (during the season) in the Elmatama area. This cross-sectional phase consisted of a parasitological survey and interviews with a questionnaire that included questions regarding sociodemographic variables, health status, health-seeking behaviour and accessibility.

One hundred (100) households (500–700 individuals) were randomly selected in each hyperendemic area. A total of 522 and 421 household members in the Malakal area and in the Elrank area, respectively, were randomly selected for the cross-sectional survey in the hypo-mesoendemic areas.

Individuals living in households that had been randomly selected for the cross-sectional phase were encouraged to report to health facilities in their catchment area in case of any febrile illness during the study period. In the follow-up phase, the records from these health facilities within the catchment areas (the cross-sectional survey area) where malaria cases had been registered were used by the study team on a monthly basis.

Main study findings

Cross-sectional phase

Within households in the hyperendemic areas, 522 and 421 individuals were interviewed in the Malakal and Elrank areas, respectively. In the hypo-mesoendemic areas, 1049 and 1636 individuals were interviewed in the Elhosh and Elmatama areas, respectively.

The prevalence of parasitaemia, fever and confirmed malaria at the time of the survey was found to be 3.3%, 21.6% and 13.0%, respectively, in the Malakal area and 0.95%, 16.2% and 5.0%, respectively, in the Elrank area. The prevalence of parasitaemia, fever and confirmed malaria at the time of the survey was found to be 1.9%, 13.3% and 3.8%, respectively, in the Elhosh area and 0.1%, 6.0% and 2.8%, respectively, in the Elmatama area.

Follow-up phase

Among 3298 patients who visited the outpatient clinics in the Malakal area, a total of 980 (29.7%) were positive, while in the Elrank area a total of 3526 (53.6) out of 6579 patients visiting outpatient clinics were positive. The incidence of malaria episodes during the follow-up period was estimated to be 8.5 (980/125 901) and 178.6 (3526/47 384) per 1000 population in the Malakal area (11 months) and the Elrank area (5 months), respectively.

In the Elhosh area, a total of 2970 (67.8%) were positive among 4382 patients who visited the outpatient clinics, while in the Elmatama area a total of 482 out of 1543 (31.2%) were positive. The incidence of malaria episodes during the follow-up period was estimated to be 23.7 (2970/150 430) and 10.3 (482/80 000) per 1000 population in the Elhosh (10 months) and Elmatama (7 months) areas, respectively.

Burden estimate

Using the prediction equation, the relationship between malaria incidence and the product of symptomatic and asymptomatic ratio (S/AS) ratio and prevalence was studied in the different areas and plotted. The best-fit model was the exponential fit, which explained 82% of the variability in the incidence (R^2 = 82%). The product of prevalence and S/AS ratio was used, based on the fact that the prevalence of confirmed symptomatic malaria cannot alone explain the pool of "infected" carriers in the community. The actual pool consists of symptomatic and asymptomatic individuals. Obtaining the ratio between symptomatic to asymptomatic indicates the "factor" by which the prevalence should be multiplied in order to obtain the true prevalence of infection, which is the main determinant of future malaria episodes in the area. In fact, the product of the S/AS ratio and prevalence explained 82% of the variability in the incidence and no other variables reported such a significant association with the incidence using multivariate logistic regression analysis.

Based on the above, the equation predicting malaria incidence (episodes/1000 population) is as follows:

Incidence = 5.8094 exp (0.1238) X
Where the slope "b" = 0.1238
And the intercept = 5.8094
X = number of years.

Using this equation, and the nationwide figures reported by the Global Fund for HIV/AIDS, Malaria and TB survey in 2006:

Prevalence of confirmed symptomatic malaria = 5.4%
Prevalence of asymptomatic parasitaemia = 2%
S/AS ratio = 2.7
Product between prevalence of symptomatic parasitaemia and S/AS ratio = 5.4 × 2.7 = 14.7.

Therefore, the incidence of malaria episodes was estimated at 35.8 (32.3–39.4) per 1000 population. With a population of 34 840 426, this will be equal to 1 249 021 episodes per year in Sudan.

Conclusions and recommendations

Using the above prediction equation will allow estimation of the incidence of malaria episodes in the future, based on the results of prevalence surveys in hypo-mesoendemic and hyperendemic areas.

Malaria

Insecticide resistance and knockdown resistance alleles in the malaria vector *Anopheles arabiensis* from eastern Sudan

- **Sudan**
  Eastern Sudan
- **Study period**
  November–December 2005

- **Small Grants Scheme**
  (SGS) 2005 No. 83

- **Principal Investigator**
  Yousif E Himeidan
  Faculty of Agriculture and Natural Resources
  University of Kassala
  New Halfa, Sudan
  e-mail: yosifhimeidan@yahoo.com

Abstract

Resistance bioassays and molecular detection of knockdown resistance (*kdr*) alleles were conducted in three populations of *Anopheles arabiensis* from eastern Sudan.

Results Mortality rates against 4% dichlorodiphenyltrichloroethane (DDT) and 1% permethrin ranged from 96.9% to 99.6% and from 98.4% to 100%, respectively. Regardless of insecticide-resistance phenotype, the overall frequencies of heterozygous L1014F and L1014S kdr alleles together were 7.0% in Kassala, 5.1% in El-Girba and 2.2% in New Halfa. A higher frequency (67%) of L1014F-*kdr* alleles associated with resistance phenotype against DDT was found in New Halfa, a cotton-growing area. More importantly, L1014S-*kdr* alleles were detected in four susceptible individuals from Kassala, where insecticide-treated nets (INTs) were used for vector control.

Conclusion Although current frequencies of *kdr* alleles are low in this study, there are concerns about the origin and spread of *kdr* alleles in *An. arabiensis* populations from Sudan.

Background

In Africa, knockdown resistance alleles (*kdr*) in malaria-vector mosquitoes have become a major problem for malaria interventions since pyrethroids are the main vector-control strategy. The first *kdr* allele observed in *Anopheles gambiae* complex was caused by a leucine–phenylalanine substitution at position 1014 of the sodium-channel gene. This allele, termed L1014F, is widespread in the S molecular form *An. gambiae s.s.* in western Africa populations and has recently been observed in east Africa. The M form of L1014F is thought to have arisen through introgression from the S form, but its occurrence is new and independent in *An. arabiensis*. Another *kdr* allele, L1014S, caused by a serine replacement at the same position, was initially identified in eastern Africa and has been found in parts of central Africa. This L1014S allele was observed recently in *An. arabiensis* from Kenya and Uganda, while the L1014F allele was observed at low frequency in *An. arabiensis* populations from the United Republic of Tanzania. It is unknown whether these are de novo mutations in *An. arabiensis* or whether they have arisen

Conclusions and implications of the study

- The L1014F allele was the predominant knockdown-resistance allele in an *An. arabiensis* population from eastern Sudan. It is possible that *An. arabiensis* in Sudan was more influenced by gene flow from west Africa.
- The L1014F allele was the only one found to be associated with the insecticide-resistant phenotype. This was the first observation for the presence of L1014F allele in a heterozygous state in resistant (live) individuals of *An. arabiensis* against the bioassay. However, the homozygous genotype of this allele, detected in eight resistant individuals to DDT from a colony established in central Sudan, could not alone explain the full expression of the resistance phenotype.
- All *kdr* alleles observed before were found in a heterozygous state, but none was correlated with resistant phenotypes. The highest frequency (67%) of the phenotypic *kdr* resistance against DDT was found in the cotton-growing area of New Halfa. In west Africa, the spread of L1014F alleles was attributed to the heavy use of DDT in the 1960s. This is also likely to be the situation in this study area. The highest level of resistance in *An. arabiensis* to DDT in Sudan was reported in the same area following the extensive use of DDT in the 1960s.
- The presence of the L1014S allele in only four susceptible individuals from Kassala could be related to the possible poor indication of the kdr L1014S allele to phenotypic (behavioural or physiological) resistance. On the other hand, this area received a large number of ITNs, distributed by the National Malaria Control Programme after the devastating floods in 2003. Perhaps the presence of the two *kdr* alleles in this area at detectable frequencies was an effect of ITN use, as in western Kenya, pyrethroid resistance was reported initially in the context of ITN use. Considering the current mortality levels with permethrin, the results suggest that vector control, rather than agricultural spraying, is the main source of selection resistance. Thus, implementation of indoor residual spraying of DDT should be reconsidered.

through introgression from *An. gambiae s.s.* Here, we report both *kdr* alleles in a heterozygous state and the presence of the L1014F allele for the first time in resistant individuals of *An. arabiensis* populations from eastern Sudan.

Materials and methods

Study area and field sampling

Cross-sectional larval surveys were conducted in the cool dry season during November and December 2005. Anopheline larvae were collected, using a standard dipper, from eight sites in three areas with different patterns of insecticide usage: (1) New Halfa (35° 20'E and 15° 34'N), an area where agriculture insecticide usage is mainly for cotton pests and indoor residual spraying is the main method to control the malaria vector; (2) El-Girba (35° 57'E and 14° 58'N), an area adjacent to the cotton area and where indoor residual spraying and larvicides are the major vector-control methods; and (3) Kassala (36° 26'E and 15° 23'N), a horticultural area located along the valley of El-Gash River, where larvicides and insecticide-treated nets (ITNs) are used for vector control.

Dichlorodiphenyltrichloroethane (DDT) was used extensively for malaria-vector control and agriculture in the 1960s, when the New Halfa agricultural scheme was established for new immigrants from northern Sudan. By the early 1980s, organophosphates and pyrethroids had replaced DDT as a consequence of insecticide resistance. These two classes of insecticides are the main compounds currently used for vector control.

Laboratory techniques

The field-collected anopheline larvae, found only in pools resulting from leaks in pipe-water supplies, were transfered into the insectary, reared to adults and morphologically identified. Insecticide bioassays were performed on non-blood-fed female adults at 1–3 days old, using WHO test tubes and protocols [1]. The insecticides tested were 4% DDT and 1% permethrin.

DNA was extracted individually from the bioassay-tested *An. arabiensis* mosquitoes, which were molecularly identified afterwards. Individual mosquitoes were screened for L1014F- and L1014S-*kdr* alleles on a Li-Cor 4300 DNA analyser, using the modified diagnostic method of Tripet et al.[2]. The positive samples for *kdr* alleles were confirmed by DNA sequencing of ~300 bp fragments amplified by primers AgD1 and AgD2.

Main study findings

The mortality rates at 24 hours postexposure and the knockdown time thresholds (KdT50 and KdT90) ranged from 96.9% to 99.6% and from 98.4% to 100% against 4% DDT and 1% permethrin, respectively. For both insecticides, there was no significant difference among the three populations (for DDT, $chi^2 = 3.83$, $df = 2$, $P = 0.15$; for permethrin, $chi^2 = 2.38$, $df = 2$, $P = 0.30$).

An. arabiensis was the only member of the *An. gambiae* complex found in the study area, consistent with previous cytogenetic results. Among 498 genotyped mosquitoes, 25 were positive for *kdr* alleles. Both *kdr* alleles (L1014F and L1014S) were detected in *kdr*/susceptible-type heterozygosities in the vector *An. arabiensis*. Regardless of insecticide-resistant phenotype, the overall *kdr* allelic frequencies were 7.0%, 5.1% and 2.2% in Kassala, El-Girba and New Halfa populations, respectively, with no significant difference in the frequencies among the three populations ($chi^2 = 4.23$, $df = 2$, $P = 0.12$). However, 84% ($n = 21$) of the kdr-alleles observed were L1014F, the predominant allele in west Africa. The frequencies of the heterozygotes with L1014F among the individuals resistant to DDT were 25%, 33% and 67% in Kassala, El-Girba and New Halfa, respectively. The L1014S allele was only detected in four susceptible individuals from Kassala.

Conclusions and recommendations

Although current frequencies of *kdr* alleles are low in this study, there are concerns about the origin and spread of *kdr* alleles in *An. arabiensis* populations from Sudan. While *kdr* alleles were first documented in *An. arabiensis* from west Africa, their detection in *An. arabiensis* from Kenya, Uganda and the United Republic of Tanzania emphasizes the need to develop appropriate strategies to manage resistance development within malaria-vector populations.

The mortality rate from DDT in New Halfa was similar to that observed by Himiedan et al. [3], indicating that there was no detectable increase in mosquito resistance over the 6-year period between the two observations.

References

[1] *Test procedures for insecticide resistance monitoring in malaria vectors, bio-efficacy and persistence of insecticides on treated surfaces. Report of the WHO Informal Consultation.* Geneva, World Health Organization, 1998.

[2] Tripet F, Wright J, Lanzaro G. A new high-performance PCR diagnostic for the detection of pyrthroid knockdown resistance kdr in *Anopheles gambiae. American Journal of Tropical Medicine and Hygiene*, 2006, 74:658–662.

[3] Himiedan YE et al. *Anopheles arabiensis* and insecticide resistance in an irrigated area of eastern Sudan. *Eastern Mediterranean Health Journal*, 2004, 10:167–174.

Malaria

Assessing knowledge, attitudes and practices regarding malaria in high-endemic districts of Balochistan, Pakistan

- **Pakistan**
  Balochistan province
- **Study period**
  November 2005–November 2006
- **Small Grants Scheme**
  (SGS) 2005 No. 78

- **Principal Investigator**
  Mehmood Sultan Paracha
  Malaria Control Programme
  Health Directorate
  Balochistan, Pakistan
  e-mail: mehmood_paracha@hotmail.com

Abstract

The aim of the study was to evaluate the knowledge, attitudes and practices of the population regarding malaria and its protective measures. The study was conducted in Panjgur, Kech and Gawadar districts in Balochistan province. Twenty-four (24) households were visited from each of the clusters and 216 questionnaires were completed by local surveyors. In addition, 77 health-care providers were interviewed to evaluate their knowledge and adherence to guidelines.

Results More than 90% of respondents knew that malaria was transmitted by mosquito bites, 85.2% of respondents said that malaria was seen in their area during summer, 59.7% recognized its transmission during monsoon and 64% of households had at least one case of malaria during the past 6 months. For 78%, the first health-care-seeking behaviour was to report to a government health facility, while 19% initially went to a private health facility.

Protective measures used against malaria were bednets (78.6%), followed by closing doors and windows and using insecticides (nearly 40% each), and keeping surroundings clean (35%). The main reason cited for using bednets was avoiding mosquito nuisance (65.7%), followed by protection from malaria (63.3%). Only 18% said that they used insecticide-treated bednets (ITNs). Evaluation of case-management practices of health-care providers found several malpractices regarding prescription of first-line drug, drug dosage and actions to be taken with severe malaria.

Conclusion The study provided baseline information regarding the knowledge of the community about malaria and its protective measures, and the extent of adherence of health-care providers to guidelines. The study identified several areas that should be targeted by future interventions.

Background

The study was conducted in Panjgur, Kech and Gawadar districts in Balochistan province. The household survey involved 14 interviewers from Panjgur district (six males and eight female), 12 from Kech district (six males and six females) and 13 from Gawadar (seven males and six females). In each district, three teams were formed comprising of one/two male and one/two female interviewers. Each team was supervised. The principal investigator and two coinvestigators were involved in supervision and monitoring field activities. Stratified cluster sampling was used to select urban and rural localities within each district; 24 households from each cluster were then visited. The entire population of the sampled households was 2611, and of these 216 were interviewed (108 males and 108 females). The total number of children under 5 years old in these families was 771 (29.5% of total). The questionnaires was completed by local surveyors.

The aim of the study was to evaluate the knowledge, attitudes and practices of the population regarding malaria and its protective measures. In addition, 77 health-care providers were interviewed in order to evaluate their knowledge and adherence to guidelines.

Conclusions and implications of the study

- Pictorial leaflets showing preventive measures and general guidelines on malaria should be distributed in the community.
- To increase community awareness of malaria and its management, health-education campaigns should also be designed for television/radio in local languages.
- The use of ITNs should be promoted by mass media campaigns.
- Public/private partnership should be established to ensure the community is kept informed about new approaches to malaria control. Mechanisms involving NGOs in malaria-control activities should be developed.
- Health-care providers at different levels, including private practitioners, should be educated about malaria, its prevention, treatment and control.
- Improving microscopy facilities for malaria diagnosis would help to ensure prompt diagnosis and treatment.

Main study findings

The mean age of the male respondents was 35.2 years compared with 30.4 years for females. Half of respondents were illiterate; of these, 63% were female and 37% were male. Most of the respondents (> 75%) slept in the open air during the summer season.

Nearly half of respondents thought that malaria was the biggest health problem in their community. However, when further prompted to choose health problems commonly found in their area from a list of diseases, flu was ranked first (93%), followed by malaria (89.8%). Regarding the source of their knowledge about malaria, 31% said it was television, while the others included from a friend or spouse, a poster or radio.

More than 90% of respondents correctly mentioned that malaria was transmitted through mosquito bites, 85.2% said that malaria was seen in their area during summer, and 59.7% were aware of its transmission during monsoon. More than half of the respondents knew that the high-risk groups for malaria infection were the under-5s and pregnant women. Only 66% mentioned that the disease could be fatal, and 47% had witnessed a death due to malaria. In the previous 6 months, 64% of the households had at least one case of malaria. The most common initial health-care seeking behaviour was to report to a government health facility (78%), followed by a private health facility (19%).

Protective measures used against malaria were bednets (78.6%), followed by closing doors and windows and using insecticides (nearly 40% each) and keeping surrounding cleans (35%); only 18% said that they used insecticide-treated bednets (ITNs). The main reasons cited for using bednets was to avoid mosquito nuisance (65.7%), followed by protection from malaria (63.3%). Of the households, 37.9% had mosquito nets for all beds, 31.8% had nets for some beds while the rest had no nets. Nearly 70% of respondents said that ordinary bednets were available at general stores while some also mentioned other sources such as nongovernmental organizations (NGOs) (10%), medical stores (10%), private hospitals (3%) or public-health facilities (5%). The average price paid for a bednet was almost US$ 6. More than 70% of respondents mentioned that bednets were expensive. About 40% were aware of ITNs and 18% said that they already had one. These responses may reflect the fact that NGOs and some health facilities had promoted ITNs. The cost they were willing to pay for an ITN ranged from less than US$ 1 to US$ 10.

Knowledge of health-care providers

Most (85.7%) health-care providers were aware that severe malaria was caused by *Plasmodium falciparum*. More than 70% recognized the two high-risk groups were under-5 children and pregnant women, but mine labourers were recognized by only 12%.

Regarding diagnosis, 75% correctly recognized that clinical malaria was diagnosed on clinical features as headache, fever, chills and vomiting. However, almost 50% failed to recognize any of the common clinical features of severe malaria. Also, 65% of respondents correctly mentioned that clinical malaria was diagnosed without microscopy and that severe malaria was confirmed by microscopic examination of blood.

With respect to management, 66% were aware of the protocol for management of severe malaria at the primary health-care facility level and the rest said cases should be referred to a higher centre without any intervention.

Although 78% said that drug of choice for treating cerebral malaria was quinine, only 18.2% knew that the loading dose of quinine was 20 mg salt/kg of body weight orally/IM/IV. In addition, 29% said patients should be treated as comatose patients, 18% mentioned blood transfusions and 23.4% mentioned corticosteroids, which are contraindicated in such patients. However, for treatment of convulsions related to cerebral malaria, 73% of respondents correctly mentioned intravenous diazepam. Nearly 86% were aware of treatment of *P. vivax* malaria by chloroquine, but only 29% further added primaquine, which is necessary to prevent relapse. Only 46% of respondents were aware that chemoprophylaxis within the country has been abandoned according to national guidelines and is not recommended in Pakistan.

Around half of respondents said posters were their main source of information regarding malaria, while 43% of respondents gave television and 41% gave radio as their source of information regarding malaria.

Conclusions and recommendations

The study provided baseline information about the knowledge of the community concerning malaria and its protective measures, and the extent of adherence of health-care providers to guidelines. The study identified several areas that should be targeted in future interventions.

Malaria

Knowledge, attitudes and practices regarding malaria in Iranshahr area, Sistan-Baluchistan Province, south-east Islamic Republic of Iran

- **Islamic Republic of Iran**
  Sistan-Baluchistan Province
- **Study period**
  2005–2006
- **Small Grants Scheme**
  (SGS) 2005 No. 232

- **Principal Investigator**
  Hamid Reza Basseri
  Department of Medical Entomology
  School of Public Health and Insititute of Public Health
  Tehran University of Medical Sciences
  Tehran, Islamic Republic of Iran
  e-mail: hamid_basseri@hotmail.com

Abstract

The study aimed at evaluating the knowledge, attitudes and practices among Afghani refugees compared with Iranian residents in Iranshahr area, Sistan-Bluchistan Province, where malaria is highly endemic. A total of 770 consenting participants, 381 Iranian and 389 Afghani refugees seeking care at the primary health care system, were interviewed about their knowledge, attitudes and practices regarding malaria, using a structured questionnaire.

Results The results revealed that most Iranians (76.6%) and Afghanis (60.1%) were familiar with the symptoms of the disease. About 52.4% of Iranians and 47.6% of Afghanis said that malaria transmission occurred by mosquito bites. About 94.6% of Afghanis had no idea about the cause of malaria, compared with 5.4% of Iranians. The study showed that a limited number of Afghani refugees seek care at the health centres. The majority of Afghanis (about 71%) did not take any measures to protect themselves against malaria transmission, while the majority of Iranians (70.3%) did. In total, 45% of all responders did not use any measures to protect themselves. The majority of Afghanis (61.2%) did not know that malaria transmission could be controlled. Around 96% of respondents agreed that malaria is a curable disease but the majority had poor knowledge about antimalarial drugs.

Conclusion Afghani refugees had a significantly lower level of knowledge regarding malaria, its mode of transmission, protective measures and types of antimalarial drugs. Increasing awareness of the population in high-endemic areas, with emphasis on Afghani refugees, is recommended.

Background

An estimated 378 000 refugees are living in Sistan-Baluchistan Province in the south-eastern Islamic Republic of Iran. The Islamic Republic of Iran borders Afghanistan and Pakistan, where malaria is still one of the major health problems. Vector insecticide and parasite drug resistance in this area has hampered malaria control. According to recent reports from the Ministry of Health in the Islamic Republic of Iran, about 24% of all malaria cases in the country in 2004 were non-Iranian and mostly Afghani refugees. During 2005, more than 59% of all cases of malaria in the country have been reported from Sistan-Bluchistan province and 24% of all cases were non-Iranians cases. This study aimed at evaluating the knowledge, attitudes and practices of Afghani refugees and comparing these with Iranian residents in a high-malaria-endemic area.

Materials and methods

The study was conducted in Iranshahr area, Sistan-Baluchistan Province, where malaria is highly endemic. At present, malaria-control programmes are undertaken by primary health care systems, consisting of health centres and health houses in rural and urban areas. A total of 770 consenting participants, 381 Iranian and 389 Afghani refugees, seeking care at the primary health care systems were interviewed about their knowledge, attitudes and practices regarding malaria, using a structured questionnaire.

Conclusions and implications of the study

- Although a considerable proportion of participants in both groups had good knowledge about the cause of malaria and the role of mosquitoes in its transmission, few participants used bednets or other protective measures.
- There is a need to increase community awareness about malaria, its protective measures and the importance of early diagnosis, timely treatment and adherence to treatment.
- An awareness programme should be developed, aimed at Afghani refugees, to increase their use of protective measures, improve their health-care seeking behaviour and increase their use of free health services in health centres. Afghanis in the area could volunteer in such awareness programmes to help increase malaria protection and prevention in the Afghani refugee community.

Main study findings

The results revealed that most Iranians (76.6%) and Afghanis (60.1%) were familiar with typical symptoms of the disease. About 52.4% of Iranian and 47.6% of Afghanis said that malaria transmission occurred by mosquito bites. About 94.6% of Afghanis had no idea about the cause of malaria, compared with 5.4% of Iranians. Health services played a strong role in increasing knowledge of Iranian residents but not for Afghani refugees. The study showed that a limited proportion of Afghanis seek care at health centres. The majority of Afghanis (about 71%) did not take any measures to protect themselves against malaria transmission, while the majority of Iranians (70.3%) used protective measures. Generally, 45% of total responders did not use anything to protect themselves. The majority of Afghanis (61.2%) did not know that malaria transmission could be controlled. However, a large number of respondents (about 96%) agreed that malaria was a curable disease. Overall, 61.4% of all participants did not know about antimalarial drugs (57.6% of Iranians and 65.1% of Afghanis).

Almost all participants (94.9%) had no mosquito nets at home and 78.3% did not use screens for windows and doors. Regarding treatment, 60.8% of all respondents had access to health services less than half an hour from their home but only 29.8% of Afghanis attended health centres for malaria treatment.

Conclusions and recommendations

The study showed that Afghanis should be provided with adequate information about malaria in the area and its complications. Public awareness about the importance of preventing malaria should also be increased. Effective communication between health-care providers and the Afghani community would help to control malaria among Afghanis, as well as Iranians, in the endemic area.

Malaria

A midwife-based strategy to increase coverage of pregnant women with intermittent preventive treatment and insecticide-treated bednets in New Halfa, eastern Sudan

- **Sudan**
  New Halfa
- **Study period**
  July 2006–April 2007

- **Small Grants Scheme**
  (SGS) 2005 No. 39

- **Principal Investigator**
  Ishag Adam
  Faculty of Medicine
  University of Khartoum
  Khartoum, Sudan
  e-mail: ishagadam@hotmail.com

Abstract

The study aimed to evaluate the impact of involving midwives in the distribution of intermittent preventive treatment (IPT) and insecticide-treated bednets (ITNs) to pregnant women on increasing coverage of these protective measures. During July 2006, all consenting midwives in New Halfa, Sudan and all consenting pregnant women in 21 out of 176 villages in the area were interviewed. Surveys were conducted in these villages in September 2006 to explore prevalence of malaria among pregnant women and risk factors (including non-usage of ITNs and IPT). Labour-room data were gathered and placental malaria investigated using direct microscopic methods and histopathology from October 2006 to April 2007. The data collection form included information about residence, usage of ITNs and IPT. Birth weight was measured and risk factors for low birth weight were studied.

Results A total of 68 (78.2%) and 139 (82.7%) of midwives and pregnant women, respectively, were aware that mosquitoes cause malaria. However, 59 (68.6%) of the midwives and almost all (162; 98%) the pregnant women had no knowledge of IPT. During the surveys in September 2006, none of the pregnant women was found to have malaria. There were 550 singleton deliveries, 404 of them were villagers; 154 (38.1%) of these villagers reported using ITNs and 25 (6.2%) reported using IPT during pregnancy. Of 278 placentae investigated by histopathology, 89 (32.0%) showed malarial infection. Placental infections had no significant association with low birth weight or maternal anaemia.

Perceptions of causes of malaria and of its complications, treatment and prevention among midwives and pregnant women were independent of their sociodemographic characteristics (e.g. age, parity, residence and education). The mean birth weight was not significantly different between women who had used ITNs or IPT and those who had not.

Conclusion The study provided good baseline information which could be used to design a communication strategy to increase coverage of IPT and ITN. Any strategy to increase use of preventive measures needs to be sustained over a period of time.

Background

In Sudan, malaria in pregnancy is associated with maternal anaemia and low-birth-weight infants and is the main cause of maternal mortality [1,2]. It has been estimated that 75 000–200 000 infant deaths are associated with malaria infection in pregnancy. Malaria infection during pregnancy is one of the few conditions causing low birth weight that is amenable to specific intervention.

The Sudanese Federal Ministry of Health recommended intermittent preventive treatment (IPT) with sulfadoxine–pyrimethamine (SP) and insecticide-treated bednets (ITN) for pregnant women in areas of intense malaria transmission

Conclusions and implications of the study

- The interviewed midwives and pregnant women had good knowledge about malaria symptoms and the majority were aware that mosquitoes cause malaria. Of the pregnant women, 43.5% did not use ITNs; their main reasons for not using them were lack of availability and inconvenience (hot, smelly and restricted movement).
- Anaemia, miscarriage and low birth weight were mentioned as complications of malaria during pregnancy by 51.8%, 8.9% and 6.5% of the pregnant women, respectively. Around one-quarter (28.6%) of the pregnant women did not mention any complication of malaria during pregnancy.
- Although the majority of midwives and almost all of the pregnant women (98%) had no knowledge of IPT, both groups expressed substantial concern about its use during pregnancy. More than one third of midwives and pregnant women mentioned that SP was harmful and unsafe for use during pregnancy. Although the majority of women considered antimalarials to be less harmful than the effects of malaria itself on pregnancy, they did not realize the role of malaria chemoprophylaxis during pregnancy.

and irrigated areas. However, according to recent surveys, only 13% and 1.8% of pregnant Sudanese women have used IPT and ITN, respectively (Malik, personal communications).

This study aimed to evaluate the impact of involving midwives in the distribution of IPT and ITNs to pregnant women on increasing coverage of these protective measures.

Materials and methods

During July 2006, all midwives in New Halfa, Sudan and all consenting pregnant women in 21 villages out of 176 villages in the area were interviewed. A pretested structured questionnaire was administered to gather their sociodemographic characteristics. Interviews began with broad, unstructured and non-directive questions about pregnancy, delivery and health of pregnant women and gradually focused on malaria in pregnancy, its complications (including fetal complications) and treatment. Special questions were included about their perception of preventive measures (ITN and IPT) and willingness to use these preventive packages in the future. Surveys were then conducted in the villages during September 2006 to explore prevalence of malaria among pregnant women and to explore risk factors (including non-usage of ITNs and IPT).

Labour-room data were gathered and placental malaria investigated using direct microscopic methods and histopathology from October 2006 to April 2007. Data collection forms included information about residence, usage of ITNs and IPT. Birthweight was measured and risk factors for low birth weight were studied.

Main study findings

During the study period, 87 midwives and 168 pregnant women were interviewed. The mean (standard deviation, SD) of the age and parity of the pregnant women were 25.6 (9.4) years and 2.5 (2.8), respectively. A total of 68 (78.2%) and 139 (82.7%) of midwives and pregnant women, respectively, were aware that mosquitoes cause malaria; 10 (6%) of the pregnant women said they did not know the cause of malaria and 5 (3%) thought malaria was caused by stagnant water. The majority of midwives and pregnant women, 83 (94.4%) and 163 (97.1%), respectively, knew two or more symptoms related to malaria. The majority (137; 81.5%) of the pregnant women would go to the doctor if they felt unwell and had symptoms suggestive of malaria, while 15 (8.9%) would go to the midwife and the remainder (16; 9.5%) would self-medicate or said they would just eat good food. Anaemia was mentioned as a complication of malaria during pregnancy by 31 (35.6%) and 87 (51.8%) of midwives and the pregnant women, respectively. More than one quarter (27; 31%) of midwives and 15 (8.9%) pregnant women mentioned miscarriage as a complication of malaria. Low birth weight was mentioned as a complication of malaria by 24 (27.6%) and 11 (6.5%) of midwives and pregnant women, respectively. More than one quarter (48; 28.6%) of pregnant women did not mention any complication of malaria in pregnancy. Around one fifth of midwives (19; 22%), and 65 (38.7%) of pregnant women mentioned that malaria treatment was harmful to the fetus. More than two fifth (73; 43.5%) of pregnant women did not use bednets, either because they were not available (21), or because they were hot (7), nasty (1), unpleasant (18), restricted their movement (13), they were lazy (13) or they thought they would not be protective (1). Around two thirds (95; 65.5%), of pregnant women who said they had used nets had not used them the previous night.

A total of 59 (68.6%) of midwives and almost all pregnant women (162; 98%), had no knowledge of IPT. More than one third (29; 33.7%) of midwives and 14 (8%) pregnant women mentioned that SP was harmful and unsafe to use during pregnancy.

Perceptions of the causes of malaria and of its complications, treatment and prevention among midwives and pregnant women were found to be independent of sociodemographic characteristics (e.g. age, parity, residence and education).

During the surveys in September 2006, none of the pregnant women was found to have malaria. There were 550 singleton deliveries, 404 of them were villagers. Of these villagers, 154 (38.1%) had a history of using ITNs and 25 (6.2%) had a history of using IPT during pregnancy.

The mean (SD) birth weight was not significantly different between those women who used ITNs and those who did not, at 3056.8 (561.32) g versus 3020.5 (551.2) g, respectively. Likewise, the mean (SD) birth weight was not significantly different between those who used IPT and those who did not, at 3062.4 (510.5) g versus 3030.1 (558.0) g, respectively.

A total of 89 (32%) of 278 placentae showed malaria infection by histopathology examinations. Of these, 6 had active, 6 had active/chronic and 77 had chronic infections. Placental infections had no significant association with low birth weight or maternal anaemia.

Conclusions and recommendations

More effort is urgently needed through different programmes (health education, training and teaching) to raise awareness of preventive measures among the vulnerable group of pregnant women. The study provided good baseline information which could be used to design a communication strategy aiming at increasing coverage of IPT and ITNs in such a community. Any strategy to increase the use of preventive measures needs to be sustained over a period of time.

References

[1] Adam I, Khamis AH, Elbashir MI. Prevalence and risk factors for *Plasmodium falciparum* malaria in pregnant women of eastern Sudan. *Malaria Journal*, 2005, 4:18.

[2] Adam I, Khamis AH, Elbashir MI. Prevalence and risk factors for anaemia in pregnant women of eastern Sudan. *Transactions of the Royal Society of Tropical Medicine and Hygiene*, 2005, 99:739–743.

Malaria

Cost effectiveness of preseason treatment with an artemisinin-based combination and its impact on interruption of malaria transmission in eastern Sudan

- **Sudan**
  Eastern Sudan
- **Study period**
  2006–2007

- **Small Grants Scheme**
  (SGS) 2006 No. 23

- **Principal Investigator**
  Badria ElSayed
  Tropical Medicine Research Institute
  Khartoum, Sudan
  e-mail: tropmed@sudanmail.net.sd

Abstract

In the malaria-endemic countries of sub-Saharan Africa, many malaria infections are asymptomatic and the majority of *Plasmodium falciparum* cases remain untreated at subpatent level as in eastern Sudan. Therefore, treatment of subpatent parasitaemia before the transmission season could have a significant impact in reducing malaria burden in the following transmission season and be considered a cost-effective method for malaria control where transmission is seasonal. The present study aimed at studying the cost–benefit of preseason treatment with artesunate/sulfadoxine–pyrimethamine (SP) compared with artesunate/SP treatment during the transmission season, and its long-term impact on malaria transmission.

A community-based intervention study was conducted in two villages in eastern Sudan for two successive years: Eltiria, where the preseason treatment was applied (intervention), and Abunaga, where no treatment was administered (control). The study was based on three cross-sectional surveys per year; the dry-season survey for detection of subpatent parasitaemia by polymerase chain reaction (PCR), the preseason survey for treatment of PCR-positive individuals in Eltiria by artesunate/SP and then the prevalence survey during the transmission season for comparison and evaluation. Data on malaria infection during the season and cost of all inputs were collected from the two villages during the transmission season using a questionnaire. Malaria cost and preseason treatment cost were estimated and used for cost–benefit analysis.

Results Parasitaemia detected by microscopy in the dry season was very low and none of the cases was symptomatic. The difference in the percentages of subpatent parasitaemia in the intervention village between 2006 (33%) and 2007 (22.2%), before and after treatment, was highly significant. The incomplete preseason treatment coverage in the intervention village in 2006 led to insignificant difference in malaria prevalence between the villages ($P > 0.05$) whereas the 100% coverage in 2007 led to zero prevalence in the intervention village during the transmission season, i.e. malaria has been completely eliminated from the village and the difference from the control village was highly significant ($P < 0.001$). The benefit ratio was 4, indicating that the cost of malaria infection during the transmission season was four times the cost of preseason treatment of subpatent carriers.

Conclusion The highly significant difference in malaria prevalence between the intervention and the control village reflects the efficiency of the treatment in elimination of malaria cases and encourages its use as an effective method of malaria control in areas of seasonal transmission.

Background

In eastern Sudan, as in other malaria-endemic countries of sub-Saharan Africa, many malaria infections are asymptomatic and the majority of *Plasmodium falciparum* infections remain at subpatent levels. Therefore, treatment of this low-level parasitaemia with artesunate/sulfadoxine–pyrimethamine (SP) before the transmission season may be considered a

Conclusions and implications of the study

- Preseason treatment with artesunate/SP for two successive years led to significant reduction in the source of infection during the dry season.
- The complete coverage of preseason treatment in 2007 had a significant impact on malaria prevalence during the transmission season and led to elimination of malaria cases in the intervention village.
- The insignificant difference in prevalence between the two villages reported in 2006 could be explained by the fact that the prevalence in the whole area was generally low due to low rainfall. Recent change of drug policy to artesunate/SP is expected to reduce the incidence of malaria according to previous findings. The treatment coverage was incomplete, missing some of the PCR-positive cases. Eltiria village was intervened for the first time and therefore the proportion of PCR positives and the prevalence during the transmission season were higher.
- A study limitation is that the proportion of transmissible subpatent parasitaemia was not evaluated. Also, no assessment was made of other factors that could have confounded the impact of the intervention.

cost-effective method for malaria control where transmission is seasonal. Successive use of this combination at this time of the year for a few consecutive years may lead to a gradual decrease in the level of the dry-season subpatent parasitaemia and hence malaria morbidity during the transmission season.

The overall objective was to study the cost effectiveness of preseason treatment of dry-season *P. falciparum* subpatent parasitaemia with artesunate/SP compared with treatment of clinical cases during the transmission season and to study the longitudinal impact of this treatment on malaria transmission.

Materials and methods

A community-based intervention study was conducted in two villages: Eltiria village, where preseason treatment was applied, and Abunaja village, where no preseason treatment was administered. The two villages were put under surveillance to collect information about the number of episodes during three transmission seasons, one baseline in 2005 and two postintervention seasons: 2006 and 2007. In 2006 and 2007, a comprehensive screening of all villagers for subpatent parasitaemia was carried out in the dry season. A finger-prick sample was collected on a glass slide for microscopic diagnosis and on filter paper for molecular analysis. Individuals who were positive by polymerase chain reaction (PCR) in June were clinically investigated and treated in August.

Before administering the first treatment dose (day 0), a drop of blood was collected on a glass slide for microscopic diagnosis and another drop on filter paper for PCR. Treatment was administered under medical supervision. Sulfadoxine–pyrimethamine (SP) was administered on day 0 as 25 mg/kg sulfadoxine/1.25 mg/kg pyrimethamine for children under 50 kg, while adults and children weighing 50 kg or more were given three tablets (each tablet contained 500 mg of sulfadoxine and 25 mg of pyrimethamine). Artesunate was given on days 0, 1 and 2 at a dose of 200 mg (two tablets at 100 mg) for adults and for children weighing 50 kg or more, while children under 50 kg received 4 mg/kg body weight. Another clinical examination was performed during the transmission season, October–November. Clinical cases were treated in the same way and malaria prevalence was estimated. The cost effectiveness of the intervention was evaluated.

Main study findings

Dry season survey (June)

The percentage of parasitaemia detected by microscopy in the two villages in June 2006 was very low (0.6%) and none of the cases was symptomatic. No case was detected positive by microscopy in the two villages during the dry season of 2007.

The percentage of subpatent parasitaemia detected by conventional PCR was significantly lower in 2007 compared with 2006 in the intervention village (22.2% and 33%, respectively).

Preseason treatment coverage in Eltiria

During the preseason of 2006, PCR was carried out for 391 persons who were present in the intervention village. Out of the 128 PCR positives, 105 were treated, 20 were absent and 3 were pregnant women. The treatment coverage in this village was 82%.

Out of 289 persons found in Eltiria during the pretransmission season of 2007, 113 were absent in the dry season. They were all tested by immunochromatographic test (ICT) and 12 of them were positive. The dry-season PCR-positive persons (50) and the ICT positives were all treated in August, i.e. the coverage was 100%.

Transmission season surveys

There was no significant difference between the intervention and control villages regarding malaria prevalence during the transmission season of 2006. However, the prevalence of malaria was significantly lower in the intervention village compared with the control village during the transmission season of 2007 (0% and 5%, respectively).

Conclusions and recommendation

The highly significant difference in malaria prevalence between the intervention and the control village reflects the efficiency of the treatment in elimination of malaria cases and encourages its use as an effective method of malaria control in areas of seasonal transmission.

Optimization protocols for testing impregnated bednets and long-lasting insecticide nets against the main malaria vector *Anopheles stephensi* in the laboratory

- **Islamic Republic of Iran**
- **Study period**
  August 2005–July 2006

- **Small Grants Scheme**
  (SGS) 2005 No. 214

- **Principal Investigator**
  Hassan Vatandoost
  School of Public Health & Institute of Health Research
  Tehran University of Medical Sciences
  Tehran, Islamic Republic of Iran
  e-mail: hvatandoost@yahoo.com

Abstract

An attempt was made to evaluate different bednets impregnated with various pyrethroids. The stability of insecticide on the bednet was measured using standard methods of washing. All tests were carried out according to WHO-recommended methods.

Results The effectiveness of bednets impregnated with permethrin, deltamethrin, bifenthrin and etofenprox was evaluated, along with the effectiveness of the long-lasting bednets Olyset Net® (polyethylene) and PermaNet® (polyester). The main malaria vector, *Anopheles stephensi*, was tested against impregnated bednets using a 3-min exposure time, and mortality was measured after a 24-h recovery period. Knock-down rate was also measured every 10 minutes. Impregnated nets showed a marked decrease in mortality of *An. stephensi* after washing, compared with unwashed nets. The only net that showed no difference in mortality with washing as reported by the tube test was the PermaNet®.

Conclusion Results of this study will be useful for WHO and local people who wish to use pyrethroid-impregnated bednets.

Background

Various methods for mosquito control have been proposed by investigators. An important innovation during the past decade has been the widespread introduction of insecticidal pyrethroid-treated mosquito nets (ITNs) for protection against transmission of vector-borne diseases, including malaria. Pyrethroids are the only insecticides recommended today for the treatment of mosquito nets due to their rapid knock-down effects and high insecticidal potency at low dosages, combined with their relative safety for human contact and domestic handling. The recommended concentration of pyrethroids depends on the texture of the net. This study aimed to evaluate the stability of bednets impregnated with various pyrethroids using standard methods of washing.

Materials and methods

Four polyester nets were 75-denier ITNs (conventionally treated with either permethrin EC (500 mg a.i./m^2), deltamethrin SC (25 mg a.i./m^2) etofenprox EW (200 mg a.i/m^2), or bifenthrin SC (25 mg a.i./m^2), by the WHO Collaborating Centre in Montpellier, France. Two additional nets were long-lasting nets: 150-denier Olyset Net® (pretreated with 1000 mg a.i./m2 permethrin) and 100-denier PermaNet® (pretreated with 55 mg a.i./m2 deltamethrin). A third net was left untreated (as negative control). Eight pieces from the same net (40 x 40 cm) were sent to each participating laboratory for cone and tube bioassays and tunnel tests before and after every washing made by the laboratory (e.g. 0x, 1x, 2x, 3x, 4x), following the WHO standard washing procedure. Non-blood-fed, 2–5-day-old susceptible female *Anopheles* mosquitoes were exposed to netting samples for 3 min, after which they were held for 24 h with access to sugar solution. Knock down was measured 60 min postexposure and mortality was measured after 24 h.

Conclusions and implications of the study

- The following bednets reported high efficacy (mortality 90–100%), which was not significantly affected by washing: PermaNet® with tube or conical methods, Olyset Net® with tube or tunnel methods, and deltamethrin with the tube method.
- The following bednets reported high efficacy, which was significantly reduced by washing: permethrin with tube, conical or tunnel methods, deltamethrin with tunnel or conical methods, Olyset Net® with the conical method, and etofenprox with the tube method.
- The remaining bednets showed a low efficacy, which was further reduced by several washings.

Main study findings

Conical tests showed a decrease in mortality rate of *Anopheles stephensi* in washed nets compared with unwashed nets for permethrin (from 90% to 67%), deltamethrin (from 99% to 70%), Olyset Net® (from 97% to 7%), PermaNet® (from 95% to 92%), bifenthrin (from 59% to 27.5%) and etofenprox (from 47.5% to 22.5%).

The mortality rate of *An. stephensi* exposed to nets impregnated with permethrin at tube tests decreased from 100% in unwashed nets to 73.3% in washed nets, while the mortality rate in washed nets decreased to 94.1% for deltamethrin, 92% for Olyset Net®, and 58% for etofenprox. The mortality decreased from 67.6% to 25% for bifenthrin, while no significant difference was detected for PermaNet®.

Results of the tunnel tests showed a decrease in mortality from 100% in unwashed nets to 7% for washed nets impregnated with permethrin, and 92% for the Olyset Net®. The decrease in mortality as shown by the tunnel test was from 94% for unwashed nets to 50% for washed nets impregnated by deltamethrin, and from 71.6% to 43.3% for nets impregnated with bifenthrin, while etofenprox showed a decrease from 87.6% to 65.5%.

Conclusions and recommendations

Pyrethroid-impregnated nets can be used for vector control of malaria in endemic areas with relative human and domestic safety. The following bednets reported high efficacy (mortality 90–100%), which was not significantly affected by washing: PermaNet® with tube or conical methods, Olyset Net® with tube or tunnel methods, and deltamethrin with the tube method.

Malaria

Efficacy of permethrin-treated plastic sheeting against malaria vectors in the south of the Islamic Republic of Iran

- **Islamic Republic of Iran**
  Baluchistan province
- **Study period**
  March 2006–February 2007
- **Small Grants Scheme**
  (SGS) 2005 No.93

- **Principal Investigator**
  Hossein Ladonni
  Department of Medical Entomology
  School of Public Health & Institute of Public Health Research
  Tehran University of Medical Sciences
  Tehran, Islamic Republic of Iran
  e-mail: ladonnih@sina.tums.ac.ir

Abstract

To evaluate the efficacy of permethrin-treated plastic sheeting (ITPS) against malaria vectors in south-east Islamic Republic of Iran, a trial was carried out in a number of small villages, each with 15–20 families.

Results Entomological evaluation commenced 5 days after ITPS application and continued at 2-week intervals in treated and untreated rooms in the selected villages. ITPS bioassay tests on adults of a laboratory and a wild strain of *Anopheles stephensi* and also on a laboratory strain of *Culex quinquefasciatus* showed a high bioefficacy, while tests on a wild strain of *Cx. tritaeniorhynchus* showed poor efficacy (0–50% mortality). Entomological indexes using hand-catch, floor-sheet and human-biting collections indoors and outdoors, indicated that ITPS was effective in reducing vector population at full coverage. Irritability tests with ITPS and permethrin-impregnated paper (0.75%) using a WHO test kit indicated that permethrin-impregnated paper was more irritant than ITPS to *An. stephensi*, whereas *Cx. tritaeniorhynchus* showed a similar irritancy response to both ITPS and permethrin-impregnated paper.

Conclusion ITPS bioassay tests on adults of a laboratory and a wild strain of *An. stephensi* and also on a laboratory strain of *Cx. quinquefasciatus* showed a high bioefficacy. Further tests on *Cx. tritaeniorhynchus* are required to optimize dosage of the insecticide on the plastic sheets.

Background

Malaria is considered to be one of the most important vector-borne diseases and is a health problem in the Islamic Republic of Iran. In 2002, the total number of malaria cases showed a 22% reduction compared with 2001, but in 2003 the number of malaria cases slightly increased, reaching around 18 000 cases. Of the total malaria cases in the country, 69% occurred in the south and south-east regions. In view of the widespread occurrence of resistance to conventional insecticide in anopheline mosquitoes, evaluation of new insecticides and regular monitoring of resistance are of high priority in vector-control programmes in the Islamic Republic of Iran. Bednets (without insecticide) are widely used by local people in the rural area of Baluchistan; therefore it seemed likely that the implementation of long-lasting permethrin-treated plastic sheeting (ITPS) in Baluchistan province would show promising results.

Materials and methods

The study area was located in the south-eastern part of the Islamic Republic of Iran, a district with a high potential for malaria transmission. The efficacy and persistence of ITPS was studied initially in the laboratory, prior to the field study. Baseline entomological parameters, ecological conditions and locations of the villages were compared. The villages were then matched into four pairs. From each pair, one village was randomly allocated either to the intervention (the ITPS

Conclusions and implications of the study

- Despite a continuous malaria-control operation implemented every year, malaria remains an important parasitic disease in the area due to various factors, including technical and administrative problems; resting behaviour of people in the transmission season; climate conditions; resistance of the main malaria vectors to insecticides; the drug resistance of the parasites; and population movement.
- In view of the widespread occurrence of resistance to conventional insecticide in anopheline mosquitoes, evaluation of some new insecticides and regular monitoring of resistance are the main priority in vector-control programmes.
- The efficacy of ITPS in decreasing numbers of mosquito populations was proved, as measured by different tests. The use of the full coverage method was most effective.

application) or the control arm. A similar method was used to select collection stations. Collection of preapplication data on vector density, night-biting catch and resting density was then carried out in the selected collecting stations before the application of ITPS.

The ITPS were applied in the selected villages as follows: (1) covering only 1/3 of the upper side of the walls versus control (sheet without insecticide), with total coverage of 72%; (2) covering only the ceiling with two strips, like a cross (X) versus control, with total coverage of 83%; (3) covering the whole room versus control, with total coverage of 36%.

The efficacy of ITPS was evaluated by different testing methods. The bioassay contact mortality test, irritability test with permethrin-impregnated papers and ITPS sheet were carried out against wild strains of *An. stephensi* and *Cx. tritaeniorhynchus*. Floor sheet collection was also carried out.

Main study findings

In untreated villages, the density of *Anopheles* and *Culex* was 48.7–62.5 and 25.5–39.5, respectively, for more than 4 months. In the village treated with ITPS covering 1/3 of the upper side of the walls (i.e. one strip per wall), 140 days of ITPS application did not show any marked decrease in the population density of mosquitoes. In the village treated with ITPS sheets at the ceiling (X shape), there was no marked decrease in population density of mosquitoes even after 140 days, with 8.8–23.1% and 9.5–23.8% mortality recorded for *Anopheles* and *Culex*, respectively. In the village treated with ITPS sheets at full coverage, a marked decrease in the density of *Anopheles* and *Culex* (4.5% and 15.2% respectively) was recorded, with a postmortality index of 0–50% and 25.8–45% for *Anopheles* and *Culex*, respectively.

A man-biting collection was made to estimate the effect of ITPS on feeding behaviour of mosquitoes in treated and untreated villages from indoors and outdoors. In untreated villages and in the two villages treated either with ITPS at one strip per wall or with two ceiling strips in an X shape, there was no remarkable decrease in population density of mosquitoes per man from indoors and outdoors. On the other hand, in villages treated with ITPS sheets at full coverage, there was a marked effect on indoor and outdoor mosquito population density.

Floor-sheet collection was made to estimate the efficacy of ITPS on resting density of mosquitoes in treated and untreated villages. In treated villages, *Anopheles* and *Culex* density decreased after 140 days. The decrease was relatively higher in the village treated with full coverage.

The result of the bioassay tests on wild strains indicated that the ITPS has a remarkable effect on *An. stephensi*, with 100% mortality recorded after 140 days of ITPS application. *Cx. tritaeniorhnchus* showed a lower response to ITPS, with 0–50% mortality recorded after 140 days of ITPS application. Permethrin-impregnated paper was more irritant than ITPS for *An. stephensi* ($P < 0.05$), while permethrin-impregnated paper and ITPS had similar irritancy for *Cx. tritaeniorhynchus* ($P > 0.05$).

Conclusions and recommendations

The efficacy of ITPS was proved to decrease the number of mosquito population as measured by different tests. The use of full coverage methods was more effective and led to a remarkable decrease in the mosquito population density in the villages studied.

Meningitis

Strengthening the rapid diagnosis and epidemiological investigation of bacterial meningitis due to *Neisseria meningitidis, Haemophilus influenzae* type b and *Streptococcus pneumoniae* using the polymerase chain reaction method

- **Tunisia**
  Tunis
- **Study period**
  2005–2006

- **Small Grants Scheme**
  (SGS) 2005 No. 147

- **Principal Investigator**
  Amal Kechrid
  Microbiology and Paediatric Unit
  Faculty of Medicine of Tunis
  Tunis, Tunisia
  e-mail: amel.kechrid@rns.tn

Abstract

A study was conducted in Tunis in 2006 to introduce the polymerase chain reaction (PCR) technique as a tool for early and specific diagnosis of bacterial meningitis and to study the validity of this method. The study also aimed to specify the specific bacterial causes along with their antigenic properties and serotype. Eighty-three (83) cerebrospinal fluid (CSF) samples were examined by conventional clinical microbiological methods and categorized into four categories: I, culture-positive CSF; II, culture-negative CSF, direct smear and/or antigen positive; III, culture-negative CSF, direct smear and/or antigen negative, however CSF were abnormal (> 100 white cells (WC)/mm^3); IV, CFS culture, direct smear and antigen detection all negative with low WC count. All CSF samples were then tested by PCR and a comparison was done to determine the sensitivity and specificity of the PCR test.

Results PCR tested positive in 14 cases (10 cases of *Neisseria meningitidis* and 4 cases of *Streptococcus pneumoniae*). Of 10 culture-positive CSF specimens (category I), 8 tested positive by PCR. Two culture-positive CSF specimens (*S. pneumoniae*) tested negative by PCR. PCR tested positive in 5 of 7 cases from category II, and 1 case in category III and none in category IV. Sensitivity and specificity were calculated as 86.6% and 98.6%, respectively.

Conclusion The results show that, although PCR had good specificity (98.6%), the sensitivity of the test was only 86.6%, which means that it would be good for confirming a diagnosis but not for detecting cases.

Background

Bacterial identification was performed using conventional methods. Microbiological examination of the cerebrospinal fluid (CSF) was performed by determining the aspect, cell count, Gram staining, direct antigen detection and culture. Serogrouping of *Neisseria meningitidis* and serotyping of *Haemophilus influenzae* (Difco™) were performed by slide agglutination using specific antisera. Detection of β-lactamase production was determined by cefinase disc (bioMérieux). Antimicrobial susceptibility was determined according to the French expert guidelines (CA-SFM 2004).

Materials and methods

Eighty three (83) CSF samples were collected and tested using conventional methods for bacterial identification in CSF. According to the results, the samples were categorized into four categories: I: culture-positive CSF; II, culture-negative CSF, direct smear and/or antigen positive; III, culture-negative CSF, direct smear and/or antigen negative, however CSF were abnormal (> 100 white cell (WC)/mm^3); IV, CFS culture, direct smear and antigen detection all negative with low WC count. All 83 samples were retested using PCR and results were compared to determine the sensitivity and specificity of the test.

Main study findings

Almost two thirds (63%) of the cases of bacterial meningitis were due to *N. meningitidis* and *Streptococcus pneumoniae*. About half of the *S. pneumoniae* strains had

Conclusions and implications of the study

- Almost two thirds (63%) of the cases of bacterial meningitis were due to *N. meningitidis* and *S. pneumoniae*.
- All *N. meningitidis* strains were susceptible to cefotaxim and to rifampin. More than half (55%) of the *N. meningitidis* strains were group B, followed by group A (31%) and C (13.8%).
- PCR is a reliable and rapid diagnostic tool for the identification of bacterial causes of culture-negative CSF. The sensitivity and specificity of PCR were 86.6% and 98.6%, respectively, compared with the gold standard. PCR is good for confirming a diagnosis but not for detecting one.

reduced susceptibility to penicillin and had intermediate reduced susceptibility to amoxicillin and cefotaxim of 10.8% and 5%, respectively.

A total of 93% of the *N. meningitidis* strains had decreased susceptibility to penicillin G (minimum inhibitory concentration (MIC) ≥ 0.12 µg/ml) and 35% to amoxicillin (MIC ≥ 0.25 µg/ml). All *N. meningitidis* strains were susceptible to cefotaxim and to rifampin. More than half (55%) the *N. meningitidis* strains were group B, followed by group A (31%) and group C (13.8%).

The sensitivity and specificity of PCR were 86.6% and 98.6%, respectively, compared with the gold standard.

Conclusions and recommendations

PCR is a reliable and rapid diagnostic tool for the identification of bacterial causes of culture-negative CSF. The sensitivity and specificity of PCR were 86.6% and 98.6%, respectively, compared with the gold standard. PCR is good for confirming a diagnosis but not for detecting one.

Meningitis

Temporal and spatial determinants of meningitis in the Tehran metropolitan area using a geographic information system (GIS)

- **Islamic Republic of Iran**
  Tehran
- **Study period**
  2005–2006

- **Small Grants Scheme**
  (SGS) 2005 No. 175

- **Principal Investigator**
  Alireza Mosavi-Jarrahi
  Infectious Diseases & Tropical Medicine Research Center
  Shaheed Beheshti University of Medical Sciences
  Tehran, Islamic Republic of Iran
  e-mail: alireza.mosavijarrahi@gmail.com

Abstract

A retrospective cohort study was carried out to estimate the incidence and identify the temporal and spatial determinants of meningitis in the Tehran metropolitan area of the Islamic Republic of Iran from 1996 till 2004, using a geographic information system (GIS). The spatial distribution of meningitis in the 114 subdistricts of Tehran municipality was determined using scan statistics cluster-detection technique. Temporal and spatial determinants of meningitis incidence were evaluated using Poisson regression.

Results The crude incidence of meningitis was 5.5 per 100 000 population under 15 years of age. There was a significantly higher incidence among males compare with females. The highest incidence was among children under 5 years, with a magnitude of 10.15 for males and 7.65 for females. Spatial distribution of the meningitis across the geographic boundaries of the Islamic Republic of Tehran revealed eight sets of cluster with risk ratios as high as 7. Several dependent variables were identified and multivariate analysis of the variables indicated that age, sex, season, family size, population density and other socioeconomic variables were associated with the occurrence of meningitis throughout the Tehran metropolitan area.

Conclusion The incidence of meningitis was low to moderate in the general population; however, it was slightly high in the under 5 years age group. The spatial variation across the geographic boundaries of Tehran could be explained by variations seen in the area-dependent variables.

Background

Meningitis is an important cause of morbidity and mortality in developing countries, with an estimated incidence rate of 4–15 cases per 100 000 populations per year. The epidemiology of meningitis has not been well studied in the Islamic Republic of Iran and limited information is available about the outbreaks of meningitis. One study estimated an incidence of 5 cases of meningitis per 100 000 of population under 5 years. Environmental risk factors for meningococcal infection, including social deprivation, overcrowding, passive smoking and weather conditions, have been suggested.

Social and environmental factors affect many infectious diseases. These have been documented at regional and global levels, but new geo-mapping techniques have helped to quantify the magnitude of these effects, to test hypotheses about the geographical distribution of the disease and to display environmental characteristics and disease incidence in a clear and interpretable way. The Tehran Municipality Office of Geographic Information System (TMOGIS) has developed a state-of-the-art geographical information system (GIS) covering the Tehran metropolitan area, which maintains different layers of information on socioeconomic indicators, population density, housing and other municipality attributes, as well as information on environmental factors that may affect health.

A study was therefore carried out to determine the incidence of meningitis and describe spatial and temporal determinants of meningitis in the greater Tehran municipality,

Conclusions and implications of the study

- We recommend that measures should be developed to decrease the variation seen in case reporting among the different health-service administrative bodies.
- We also recommend re-examining the reporting system, developing definitions and coding to increase the quality and quantity of data reported for each case.
- Further work is also recommended to improve the flow of data from hospitals to Ministry of Health offices of disease control.

utilizing GIS-based data layers as well as epidemiological data obtained from cases of meningitis occurring in the defined population living in the 22 districts (114 subdistricts) of Tehran municipality from 1996 till 2004. Defining the determinants of spatial and temporal distribution of the disease will improve the understanding of its epidemic features in the target population for future preventive and control measures.

Materials and methods

A retrospective cohort study evaluating the incidence and risk factors of meningitis in the Tehran metropolitan area population was carried out. All incidence cases of meningitis occurring in the target population from 1996 to 2004 that had been reported to the district health centres were included in the study. A standard case investigation procedure was performed. Abstracted cases were geo-referenced based on their residency address by the Tehran municipality GIS office. Age and sex-specific incidence was estimated for each year and 22 municipality districts of the Tehran metropolitan area. After being geo-referenced, information abstracted for each case was entered into the Microsoft Office Access database management software. Two levels of analysis were performed: descriptive and analytical using SPSS and Stata, and Epi Info, Epi Map. The spatial distribution of meningitis in the 114 subdistricts of Tehran municipality was determined using scan statistics cluster-detection technique. Temporal and spatial determinants of meningitis incidence were evaluated using Poisson regression.

Main study findings

A total of 4633 cases were recorded over the period 1996 to 2004. Data of clinical importance were available for only 2906 cases (63%). The age at onset was present for 4273 cases with a mean ± standard deviation of 17 ± 18, with a range 2 months to 93 years. More than half (56%) were children under 15 years of age. Male gender was associated with higher risk compared with female and constituted 70% of cases.

Bacterial meningitis represented more than half the cases (56%) followed by viral meningitis (16%). The highest frequency of cases (28%) occurred in spring, followed by summer, fall and winter (25.6%, 23.4% and 22.2%, respectively). The average incidence over the 7 years (1999–2005) was 3.57 (all ages combined), 5.47 for age under 15 years and 2.10 for age over 15 years, per 100 000 population.

Around eight clusters of meningitis cases over the 114 subdistrict of Tehran municipality were identified, with relative risk of clustering ranging from 1.7 to 6.8. This indicated that certain factors were in fact involved in the temporal and spatial distribution of meningitis over these years in the Tehran municipality districts.

The temporal variation of meningitis was associated with seasonal variation and showed a higher risk in spring (relative risk, RR: 1.31; 95% confidence interval, CI: 1.20–1.41) as well as in autumn (RR: 1.16, 95% CI: 1.06–1.27). Males had 2.4 times more risk for meningitis compared with female (95% CI: 2.12 and 2.41, respectively). Younger age was associated with higher risk (RR: 4.50; 95% CI: 3.97–5.09 for age group 15–50 years and RR: 8.48; 95% CI: 7.53–9.54 for age group less than 15 years).

Several dependent variables were identified and multivariate analysis of the variables indicated that age, sex, season, family size, population density and other indicators of socioeconomic variables were associated with the occurrence of meningitis throughout Tehran metropolitan area.

Conclusions and recommendations

The incidence of meningitis in our population was moderate, with a magnitude of 5.4 for age group less than 15 years. The age-specific incidence of meningitis was higher among males compared with females in all age groups. Certain area and subdistricts of Tehran were more susceptible to clustering meningitis case. Area-dependent variables were important in the distribution of meningitis cases. Further similar studies are needed to clarify the epidemiology of meningitis in the Tehran metropolitan area.

Rabies

Assessment of the burden and determinants of dog bites and public services available for victims in Lahore district, Pakistan

- **Pakistan**
  Lahore district
- **Study period**
  2005–2006
- **Small Grants Scheme**
  (SGS) 2005 No. 34

- **Principal Investigator**
  Muhammad Aslam Bajwa
  Institute of Public Health
  Lahore, Pakistan
  e-mail: aslm_71@yahoo.com

Abstract

A community-based survey was carried out to assess the burden, determinants and public services available for dog bites in Lahore district, Pakistan.

Results The prevalence of dog bites in the study population was 21.3%. The most common site of bites was the legs (68.4%), followed by the abdomen or trunk (12.1%), and hands or arms (5.6%). Among respondents to an exit interview administered to clients seeking care from an antirabies centre, the most frequent age group of victims of dog bites was 16–60 years (53.4%). The majority of respondents had been bitten by stray dogs (63), while 47 respondents were bitten by their own or others' pet dogs. Six respondents reported bites from rabid dogs. One hundred and seven (107) respondents said they had received vaccination at dog-bite centres; 89% of respondents confirmed the availability of vaccine, while 74.1% respondents said that they did not pay fees for services.

Conclusion The life-time prevalence of dog bites among respondents was 21.3%. The most frequent age group of victims of dog bites was 16–60 years. Both stray and pet dogs had bitten the victims.

Background

Pakistan, a rabies-endemic country, has no effective surveillance network to assess the magnitude of the disease. The incidence of rabies was estimated to range between 7.0 and 9.8 cases per million annually [1]. Every day, 25–30 new cases of dog bites are treated at the civil hospital in Karachi. In the absence of any accurate number of rabies deaths, a projected estimate by the Infectious Disease Society of Pakistan suggests there are around 2000–5000 rabies deaths per year [2]. The estimated prevalence of dog bites in Punjab is 0.03%, but no such estimate is available for Lahore [3]. A study in Pakistan showed that the median age of rabies cases was 22 years and that 55% of cases were aged less than 15 years. Among victims, 23% did not receive any vaccine, 67% received sheep brain vaccine (SBV) and, of these, only 40% received a full course. There was no administration of rabies immunoglobulin (RIG) or cell-culture vaccines. In-house potency testing of the vaccine batch by the manufacturer was adequate. Samples of SBV from the batch collected at the peripheral sites showed no potency.

Materials and methods

A cross-sectional community-based epidemiological study was conducted in Lahore district. The study population was a mix of urban and rural communities. The estimated sample size was 952. This sample was identified through cluster sampling, taking nine towns (clusters) in Lahore district. Interviews were then conducted in 1080 households, which was more than the estimated sample size.

Conclusions and implications of the study

- The prevalence of dog bites among respondents was 21.3%. This prevalence reflects the number of respondents ever bitten by dogs.
- The most frequent age group of victims of dog bites was 16–60 years. The second most frequent age group was 5–15 years.
- The majority of respondents were bitten by stray dogs. The most frequent site of bites was on the legs, followed by the abdomen or trunk, then the hands or arms. Six respondents reported that rabid dogs had bitten them.
- This study highlights the importance of tetanus toxoid vaccination following animal bite wounds. Only 5.4% of victims received prophylaxis against tetanus following the dog bite.
- Of these respondents, 62.2% were given vaccine at the para-umbilical region which means that two-third of victims could not choose a more-effective vaccine due to their limited purchasing power.

An exit interview was administered to clients seeking care from a dog-bite management centre. To achieve 100 interviews, every third dog-bite victim visiting the centre during the days of data collection was interviewed. Data were collected using semi-structured questionnaires in the local language. After revision, the final data were divided into four sections: consent sheet, personal profile, information about the dog bite and practices after the dog bite, and information about the pet dog.

Main study findings

The prevalence of dog bites in the study population was 21.3%. In 215 cases of dog-bite victims, 115 had been bitten by stray dogs. The most common site of bites was the legs (68.4%), followed by the abdomen or trunk (12.1%) and arms and hands (5.6%). Fifty-four (54) cases were bitten at noon or during the afternoon, followed by 34 in the morning, 24 in the evening and 21 during the night. Four respondents reported a death due to a dog bite in their families.

Regarding treatment options, 45 respondents were treated at home, while 38 went to a general practitioner, 36 to a health-care centre, eight to a hakim and six opted for a spiritual healer. Only 17.7% of respondents said that services for the management of dog bites were available in their area. Regarding the type of management received, 9.3% of respondents received wound-management services, while 2.8% received vaccination services.

It was found that 9.9% of respondents kept pet dogs; one third of those respondents had vaccinated their pet dogs.

Among the respondents to the exit interview administered to clients seeking care from the antirabies centre, the most frequent age group of victims of dog bites was 16–60 years (53.4% of respondents). Only 8.6% and 5.2% of victims belonged to age groups 0–5 years, and 60 years and above, respectively. The majority of respondents in this study were bitten by stray dogs (63), while 47 respondents were bitten by their own or others' pet dogs. Six respondents reported bites from rabid dogs.

One hundred and seven (107) respondents said they had received vaccination at a dog-bite centre, while nine respondents said that only their bite wound had been managed at the centre. A total of 89% of respondents said that vaccine had been available, while 74.1% of respondents said that they did not pay for the vaccine. Regarding the site of vaccine administration, 62.2% of respondents received vaccine at the para-umbilical region, whereas 37.8% of victims were given vaccine intramuscularly.

Conclusions and recommendations

The life-time prevalence of dog bites among respondents was 21.3%. The most frequent age group of dog-bite victims was 16–60 years. The study identified the large gap between availability of tetanus toxoid prophylaxis for road injures and following animal bites. Most respondents had to rely on nerve tissue vaccine due to limited purchasing power.

References

[1] Parviz S et al. Rabies deaths in Pakistan: results of ineffective post-exposure treatment. *International Journal of Infectious Diseases*, 2004, 8:346–352.

[2] Warrel DA, Warrel NJ. Human rabies: a continuing challenge in the tropical world. *Schweizerische Medizinische Wochenschrift*, 1995, 125:879–885.

[3] *World survey of rabies: no. 35: for the year 1999*. Geneva, World Health Organization, 2002. (WHO/CDS/CSR/EPH/2002.10).

Rabies

Evaluation of antibody response to oral rabies vaccine among wolves

- **Islamic Republic of Iran**
- **Study period**
  2006–2007

- **Small Grants Scheme**
  (SGS) 2006 No. 46

- **Principal Investigator**
  Ali Reza Janani
  Pasteur Institute of Iran
  WHO Collaborating Centre for Reference and Research on Rabies
  Tehran, Islamic Republic of Iran
  e-mail: Jananialireza@gmail.com

Abstract

Rabies is endemic in the Islamic Republic of Iran. It is the most important zoonotic disease in the country. There is evidence that the main reservoirs for rabies are wolves. Rabies incidence in man and animals is increasing each year. The main objectives of the study were to evaluate the possibility of controlling rabies in the Islamic Republic of Iran using oral vaccination of wolves and to evaluate the immune response to oral rabies vaccine among wolves.

Results The study was carried out in 1 year and 15 wolves were experimentally vaccinated using an oral rabies vaccine [Rab oral VRG (FMPB fish meal polymer bait)]. Prior to vaccination, the health status of each animal was examined. For the application of the oral rabies vaccine, the animals were anaesthetized using tranquillizers. Also a blood sample was taken to show the animals to be seronegative for rabies prior to vaccination. On days 30 and 60 after vaccination, blood samples were collected and tested for the presence of virus-neutralizing antibodies using the rapid fluorescent focus inhibition test. The animals were seropositive but the titres of neutralizing antibody were not high enough to be protective.

Conclusion The final evaluation of titres showed that the level of neutralizing antibody was not protective against natural infection, thus more studies are needed in this respect.

Background

Rabies is one of the oldest and most feared diseases of human and animals. It was recognized in Egypt before 2300 BC and in ancient Greece. The estimated annual cost of rabies in Asia is US$ 563 million [1]. Rabies is the most important zoonosis in the Islamic Republic of Iran. The rate of post-exposure prophylaxis was more than 120 000 in 2006 and the incidence of rabies is increasing each year. According to many studies during the past 50 years, the major factor for rabies in the Islamic Republic of Iran is wolves. Oral rabies vaccination of wildlife began in 1970, to reduce the cost and danger of rabies and control the disease. In this preliminary study the main idea was to evaluate the efficacy of oral rabies vaccine in wolves.

Materials and methods

The sample size was 15 wolves from three different parts of the country: eight wolves from Eram Zoo Park, 15 km from Tehran; three wolves from the Pardisan National Park in the north of Tehran and four wolves from Arak Zoo, nearly 300 km from Tehran. The study was carried out using an oral rabies vaccine [Raboral (FMPB)]. Before administration of the oral vaccine, all the animals were tested for their health status and were tranquillized using a combination of anaesthetics (ketamin 10%, 20 mg/kg and xylazine 2%, 4 mg/kg) with a gun (Telinject). Blood samples (about 2–5 ml) were taken from the brachial veins of the wolves. These samples were examined for probable neutralizing antibody. The wolves were then starved for 24 h before administration of the oral vaccine. The time taken to consume the vaccine varied, with different animals taking from 10 min to 6 h to

Conclusions and implications of the study

- The titres of the sera were too low to protect against infection. There seems to be some interfering factors. Some of these factors may relate to the animal husbandry, for example some of the wolves may not have been completely starved and thus did not accept the bait well. Another factor may have been the short period of monitoring the animals after implementation of the vaccine.
- Factors that seem to be important with oral vaccines are the size and shape of the bait; cubic and large bait is not very suitable while spherical or ovoid forms may be more applicable. Another factor is the fragility of the covering membrane, which was easily broken when thrown out.
- Storage and transportation of the vaccine may also be influencing factors.

take and chew the bait. Blood samples were taken according to the above method 1 month and 2 months later and the results obtained before and after vaccination were compared. The rapid fluorescent focus inhibition test was used for evaluation of neutralizing antibodies.

Main study findings

After seroneutralization tests on blood samples using the rapid fluorescent focus inhibition test, the level of neutralizing antibody in the wolves before oral vaccination was negligible. At 30 days after oral vaccination, a small increase of neutralizing antibody was observed in the wolves' sera. Sixty (60) days after oral vaccination the seroneutralization tests showed a trace increase in neutralizing antibody.

Comparison of the results from the first and second blood sampling did not show a significant difference among the serum titres of wolves in the study period.

Conclusions and recommendations

The final evaluation of titres showed that this level of neutralizing antibody is not protective against natural infection. To obtain more valid results, further studies are required.

References

[1] *WHO expert consultation on rabies.* First Report TRS 931. Geneva, World Health Organization, 2005.

Egypt

Schistosomiasis

Assessment of the marginal error in diagnosis of and cure from *Schistosoma mansoni* in low-endemic areas using more sensitive techniques

- **Egypt**
  Abis, Alexandria
- **Study period**
  August 2005–July 2006
- **Small Grants Scheme**
  (SGS) 2005 No. 229

- **Principal Investigator**
  Amal Farahat Allam
  Medical Research Institute
  Alexandria University
  Alexandria, Egypt
  e-mail: amalalam2005@yahoo.com

Abstract

A study was conducted to estimate the rate of false-negative results in the diagnosis of *Schistosoma mansoni* in low-endemic areas and after treatment in order to maximize the accuracy of future studies.

Results Among children with a negative diagnosis of *S. mansoni* using the Kato–Katz method, 11% and 23.3% were found to be positive using the Percoll technique and the polymerase chain reaction (PCR) method, respectively. The Percoll technique efficiently detected cases with low egg count. The Kato–Katz method gave a higher cure rate (97%) than the Percoll and PCR methods (90% and 71.4%, respectively). The PCR technique detected more positive cases than both the Kato–Katz and Percoll methods. However, the PCR gave negative results in cases diagnosed by the Percoll and Kato–Katz methods. The Kato–Katz method failed to detect eggs in very-low-intensity cases.

Conclusion A marginal error of 11% should be considered with the Kato–Katz technique as proved by the Percoll method, which should be considered the method of choice for diagnosis and post-treatment evaluation of *S. mansoni*.

Background

Consistent diagnosis of schistosomiasis still depends on coprological demonstration of schistosomiasis eggs in faecal samples. The Kato–Katz technique is currently the method of choice because of its many practical advantages in examining large numbers of people at low cost, within a short time. However, it was observed that the sensitivity of this method is less appropriate in low-endemic areas, in post-treatment situations and in determination of incidence. The Percoll technique, based on the greater density of viable schistosomiasis eggs relative to faecal matter, always gives better estimates than the conventional Kato–Katz analysis, showing less variability and detecting low-intensity infection more efficiently.

Antibody detection has been evaluated as an adjunct to faecal examination. However, cross-reactivity with other helminthes infections and low sensitivity after treatment constitute great disadvantages of immunological methods. One possible solution to this problem could be to search for circulating antigen rather than antibodies. A novel method for the detection of *Schistosoma mansoni* DNA in human samples based on the amplification of high repeated

Conclusions and implications of the study

- After a successful control programme, the epidemiological pattern of schistosomiasis has changed from high to low prevalence and low intensity in some areas in Egypt.
- A survey on 995 school children showed a prevalence of 5.7% for *S. mansoni* with 84% passing less than 100 eggs/g of faeces, indicating a low prevalence and intensity of infection.
- Among 100 negative Kato–Katz cases, 11% were shown to be *S. mansoni* positive by the Percoll technique. Of these cases, 80% passed 4 eggs/g of faeces, which indicated the efficacy of the Percoll technique in detecting cases with a low egg count.
- Among 77 negative cases by the Kato–Katz method, the PCR technique detected 18 positive cases (23%), while the Percoll technique detected 11% positive cases.
- The Kato–Katz method gave the highest cure rate (97%), followed by the Percoll and then the PCR method (90% and 71%, respectively).
- No eggs were found in faeces of 18 individuals diagnosed positive by PCR. On the other hand, PCR failed to detect 4 positive cases detected by the Kato–Katz and Percoll methods.
- The results of this study indicate that the Percoll method is the diagnostic technique of choice for the diagnosis of *S. mansoni* in low-prevalence and low-intensity areas.

DNA sequence has been developed. This test was found to be of high sensitivity and specificity. Thus, this DNA amplification assay may constitute an unprecedented alternative diagnostic technique in low-endemic areas and in light infection intensity.

Materials and methods

A cross-sectional study was carried out on primary school children in Abis 8 and 4 villages, 20 km south of Alexandria. A total of 995 stool samples were collected from the two villages, after which 156 patients received praziquantel as a single oral dose of 40 mg/kg body weight, administered on an empty stomach. One month after treatment, 105 cases submitted stool samples. All samples were examined by the Kato–Katz and Percoll methods. Seventy (70) cases were examined by the polymerase chain reaction (PCR) method. To estimate the rate of false-negative results after the Kato–Katz method, a sample of 100 students who gave negative results after Kato–Katz testing for *S. mansoni* were asked to give stool samples to be tested by both the Percoll and PCR methods.

Main study findings

Coinfection of *Schistosoma* with other parasites was found in 12.4% of cases. Among infected children, 83.9% had light infection, 10.7% had moderate and 5.4% had heavy infection. The highest egg count was found among ages 11–12 years. The prevalence of infection was higher among males. Among children with negative *S. mansoni* infection by the Kato–Katz method, 11% and 23.33% were positive by the Percoll and PCR techniques, respectively. Low egg counts were detected efficiently only by the Percoll technique (80%). By comparing the results of 77 cases studied by PCR with their results by Percoll, it was found that only 2 patients gave concordant positive results while 7 cases that were positive by Percoll were negative by PCR. Kato–Katz gave a higher cure rate (97%) than Percoll (90%) and PCR (71.4%). The PCR method detected more positive cases than both Kato–Katz and Percoll methods. However, PCR gave negative results in cases diagnosed by Percoll and Kato–Katz. The Kato–Katz method failed to detect eggs in very-low-intensity cases and overestimated the number of eggs in other case.

Conclusions

A marginal error of 11% should be considered with the Kato–Katz technique as proved by the Percoll method. False-positive and negative cases were frequently encountered with the PCR technique, compared with the results of the other two tests. Percoll may be considered the technique of choice for diagnosis and post-treatment evaluation of *S. mansoni*.

Yemen

Sexually transmitted disease

Health-seeking behaviour of sexually transmitted disease patients in Yemen

- **Yemen**
  Sana'a and Aden governorates
- **Study period**
  2006–2007

- **Small Grants Scheme**
  (SGS) 2006 No. 49

- **Principal Investigator**
  Arwa Mohammed Al-Rabee
  Department of Reproductive Health
  Ministry of Public Health and Population
  Sana'a, Yemen
  e-mail: arwaelrabee@yemen.net.ye

Abstract

A study was carried out to assess the health-seeking behaviour of sexually transmitted disease (STD) patients in Sana'a and Aden governorates of Yemen. One hundred and twenty-one (121) patients attending STD facilities at government hospitals and private facilities were enrolled and interviewed by a team of medical doctors led by a public-health expert over a 1-month period. A well-defined, pretested and WHO Regional Office for the Eastern Mediterranean-approved comprehensive and structured questionnaire was used for data collection.

Results Awareness regarding STDs was low, although it was high for HIV. The main symptoms reported by patients seeking treatment were genital discharge, lower abdominal pain and dysuria. Most STD patients first sought help from pharmacists, followed by unqualified practitioners, private clinics and, finally, private hospitals and government health institutions. There was a significant delay in seeking medical advice, mostly due to shyness. Formal communication regarding STDs through media or interpersonal approaches was low. There was also a low level of satisfaction with facilities owing to the lack of proper infrastructure and the inadequate number of qualified professionals.

Conclusion Public-awareness programmes that focus on STDs and their mode of transmission are needed. Interpersonal communication approaches should be encouraged to reduce stigma in the community and further education should be provided for health-care workers, especially pharmacists who are the first point of contact for the majority of patients.

Background

The increasing risk of HIV/AIDS among sexually transmitted disease (STD) patients emphasizes the urgent need for increased support for research and education in the prevention and control of STDs. During the past decade, many studies have provided data on the link between the HIV virus and STDs, emphasizing the importance of combating STDs in order to prevent spread of the HIV infection. Despite the awareness campaigns carried out by the Government of Yemen, STDs still have a high rate of prevalence and remain stigmatized.

Regarding seeking information about STDs, their diagnosis and prevention, an individual's behaviour is influenced by his or her perceptions, beliefs, sociocultural environment and availability of doctors and facilities. The diagnosis of STDs causes an emotional response generally unlike that of other diagnoses. A further difficulty associated with STDs is that, unlike in other medical conditions where behaviour is an individual concern, preventive health behaviour against STDs requires the co-operation of a sexual partner. Therefore, it is much more difficult to evaluate or predict safer sex practices (e.g. condom use) because of the extra person(s) involved. Strategies to assist individuals should promote self-esteem and assertiveness because often it is an individual's negotiating skills and communication with their sexual partners that is the most important factor in his or her ability to consistently follow safer sex guidelines.

Conclusions and implications of the study

- Awareness programmes focusing on STDs and their modes of transmission are required.
- Interpersonal communication approaches should be encouraged to reduce the stigma of STDs in the community.
- Pharmacists are the first point of reference for most STD patients and hence should be involved in STD/HIV programme management. This would not only result in higher curability but would also reduce the time lag between infection and treatment, thus reducing the possibility of further transmission to partners.
- Private health-care providers should be trained in STD/HIV programmes to influence health-seeking behaviour of STD patients and should refer cases to specialized government institutions to promote safe sexual practices.
- There is an urgent need to establish specialized STD clinics with comprehensive facilities in nodal cities.

Materials and methods

This was an exploratory study involving male and female patients attending STD departments in leading hospitals, and health providers treating STD patients, in Sana'a and Aden governorates. The sample consisted of 121 patients managed by 32 health-care providers, including government doctors, qualified private doctors, unqualified private practitioners and pharmacists. All patients were interviewed using a well-designed, WHO-EMRO-approved and pretested structured questionnaire to test their knowledge of STDs, their health-seeking behaviour, their perception about availability of facilities and human resources to meet their psychosocial and medical needs, and their suggestions to improve the treatment.

Main study findings

The study gave insight into patients' awareness of STDs and their methods of seeking health care. The majority of patients were aware of HIV/AIDS (88%), followed by hepatitis B (36%), gonorrhoea (33%), and syphilis and herpes simplex (28% each). Sexual intercourse (98%) and transfusion of infected blood (63%) were reported as leading modes of transmission, followed by shaving tools (37%), mother to baby transmission (11%) and infected/contaminated syringes (9%). Only 20% of respondents thought that STDs were curable. More than 75% had sought initial medical advice from a pharmacist and 12% had attended a private doctor.

The main symptoms reported by patients seeking treatment were genital discharge, lower abdominal pain and dysuria. Patients reported a lack of formal communication about STDs through the media or interpersonal approaches. They also reported a lack of proper infrastructure (agreed by practitioners) and an inadequate number of qualified professionals.

Regarding patients interviewed at government health facilities, 60% said they were satisfied with the visited health facility (public or private). Less than 50% said that they would prefer to visit a public health facility, citing "availability of services at a low price" as the main reason.

Qualified doctors, unqualified practitioners and government health professionals all agreed that buildings with specialized STD health-care facilities and the promotion of awareness campaigns were crucial for the control and treatment of STDs.

Conclusions and recommendations

Awareness programmes focusing on STDs and their mode of transmission should be increased, and interpersonal communication should be encouraged to reduce the stigma of STD in the community. For most STD patients, pharmacists were the first group approached and hence pharmacists should be involved in STD/HIV programme management. This would not only result in better treatment but would also reduce the time lag between infection and treatment, thus reducing the possibility of further transmission to partners.

Tuberculosis

Enhancing tuberculosis case detection through involving private practitioners in selected areas of Thatta district, Sindh Province, Pakistan

- **Pakistan**
  Sindh Province
- **Study period**
  April–October 2007

- **Small Grants Scheme**
  (SGS) 2005 No. 189

- **Principal Investigator**
  Zafar Fatmi
  Department of Community Health Sciences
  Aga Khan University
  Karachi, Pakistan
  e-mail: zafar.fatmi@aku.edu

Abstract

Pakistan has the highest burden (44%) of tuberculosis (TB) in the WHO Eastern Mediterranean Region and has the sixth highest burden globally. About 70% of patients seek care from private practitioners, while TB care is mainly provided by the public sector. Therefore, private practitioner involvement is an essential step in TB control. A study was conducted to enhance the case detection rate through the public–private mix (PPM) model and to review the applicability of this model in controlling TB in Thatta district, Sindh province, Pakistan.

Thatta is a rural district with a population of 1.1 million (1998 census). Of approximately 200 private practitioners, 23 were given training on DOTS. Sputum tests for patients were conducted at private laboratories and US$ 0.9 was given as an incentive to the private practitioner for identifying each TB case. The new TB cases diagnosed by private practitioners were registered with the National TB Control Programme (NTP). Anti-TB drugs were then provided by the NTP and a liaison worker from the NTP coordinated field activities. Data from the second and third quarters of 2007 were compared.

Results The total number of cases notified by public DOTS centres in the second quarter of 2007 was 186, while 211 cases were notified in the third quarter. Our intervention detected 23 new cases of sputum-smear-positive TB cases. While private laboratories were willing to do the sputum-smear testing at low cost, physicians felt that the incentives were very low.

Conclusion This study reported a workable PPM model for TB in a rural district of a developing country where private practitioners are the main health-care provider. With some amendments, it may be possible for the NTP to scale-up this model.

Background

The concept of public–private partnership has emerged in the past decade, with the realization that in many countries the public sector was not providing adequate services to large segments of the population. These partnerships between governmental and private for-profit and not-for-profit organizations have emerged in a new approach to improving the whole health-care delivery system. The need

Conclusions and implications of the study

- The study reported the feasibility of, and challenges related to, the implementation of the PPM model of collaboration between the public and private health-care sectors. The lessons learned may help in the future expansion of this PPM model in this country.
- The PPM pilot model was based on the following framework:
  - Private practitioners were responsible for recording information about the newly diagnosed sputum-smear-positive TB patients and they also sent this information monthly to the office of the district TB coordinator.
  - Private practitioners prescribed three samples of sputum smear for AFB as the main diagnostic tool for pulmonary TB. If negative, they requested X-rays for the diagnosis of sputum-smear-negative TB.
  - On request, private physians were provided with anti-TB courses from the office of the district TB coordinator in Thatta.
  - All private physiancs were given 3-monthly incentives for identification of a TB case (US$ 0.9) and the laboratory charges were paid every 2 months.
  - The field coordinator was in contact with, and coordinated, laboratory staff, private practitioners, district NTP office staff as well as the CHS-AKU team. In addition, he was responsible for retrieving information from the PPs and reporting this to the district TB coordinator.

for these partnerships was realized because the public sector was becoming overwhelmed by the burden of its service utilization and, as a result, the service it was providing was becoming inefficient and inadequate.

Currently, this partnership has received popularity under the name of public–private mix (PPM) DOTS and this model has been adopted by many countries. This PPM model of partnership has been successful in achieving international tuberculosis (TB) control targets of detecting 70% of TB cases and treating 85% of these.

The majority of the population of Thatta city, Sindh province, seeks care from private practitioners, whose case management of TB patients is generally not in line with the National TB Control Programme (NTP) guidelines. This study aimed to pilot test a PPM model in Sindh province that involved collaboration between the public sector (NTP) and private practitioners.

Materials and methods

This study was conducted in Thatta city, Thatta district, Sindh province, Pakistan, between April and October 2007.

Initially, baseline data were collected from the district TB office. About 60 private practitioners were sent a formal invitation to attend a 3-day training workshop on TB DOTS. The private practitioners were given training on TB-DOTS by the NTP master trainer. All the private practitioners were asked to complete a questionnaire based on knowledge, attitude and practices about TB and DOTS before and after the training. A total of 23 private practitioners then consented to be involved in the study after this training. These private practitioners were asked to work in partnership with the NTP and follow NTP guidelines to treat TB patients.

Main study findings

This 6-month intervention project was implemented in May 2007 and ended in October 2007. It was a pilot project and the expected outcomes of the study were to see how PPs behaved in collaboration with the government and how they practiced the standard guidelines for the management of TB.

Although participants' knowledge of managing TB cases was improved considerably, there was much overall resistance towards the PPM partnership. The 23 physicians who received training on TB-DOTS and who consented to work with the project referred a total of 55 suspected cases of TB, all of them adults.

All of these patients were sputum-smear tested for acid fast bacilli (AFB) at an assigned laboratory. The patients agreed to go for three consecutive samples of sputum smear. Of the 55 suspected cases of TB, 23 were sputum-smear positive. The TB field coordinator took the TB01 forms from the private practitioners and registered their patients with the district NTP office in Thatta. After receiving the patient profiles, the NTP office then gave the private practitioners the anti-TB treatment course. The private practitioners then gave the patients their anti-TB treatment course of drugs, initially for a period of 2 months for the intensive phase of the treatment and later for 6 months in the continuation phase. The project paid the laboratory charges for the patients' sputum AFB smear tests on a 2-monthly basis.

Every week the study field coordinator visited the private practitioners to collect their data, which was then shared with the NTP coordinator who, in turn, then revisited the private practitioners.

The project team from the Department of Community Health Sciences, Aga Khan University (CHS-AKU)) visited the private practitioners and the NTP office four times in the 6-month period between May and October 2007, while the field coordinator from the CHS-AKU team was in close liaison with the project and dealt with any issues as they arose.

A total of 23 sputum-smear-positive cases were detected during the study period. Of these, 52% (n = 12) were male and 48% (n = 11) were female. The mean age of the patients was 34 years. Most of the patients, 91% (n = 21) had no literacy. Almost half of the patients (43.5%) were workers or labourers. The majority (91%, n = 10), of the women patients were housewives.

Those who belonged to urban areas were in the majority (49%), followed by the semi-urban (about 35%) and lastly the rural (about 16%). About 24% of the patients had a family contact with TB. The monthly personal income of all patients was below 3000 rupees (US$ 50).

Case notification in Thatta district was usually below 200 each quarter year. In the first quarter of 2007 it was 202, falling to 186 in the second quarter of 2007, the period when this intervention started. The results of the intervention can be seen from the cases detected in the third quarter of 2007. The total cases notified to the NTP office in Thatta in the third quarter were 188. However, the addition of the 23 cases detected by the private practitioners who participated in this study increased the total cases in the third quarter to 211.

Conclusions and recommendations

This study reported a workable PPM model for TB in a rural district of a developing country where private practitioners are the main health-care providers. This model may be scaled-up by the NTP with some amendments. For any PPM activity, the governmental role should be of stewardship and this should be fulfilled with sincerity and responsibility to create a sense of responsibility and trust within the partnership. Any shortcomings in communication between the partners can lead to misunderstandings. In addition, it is very important that the patients, who are the prime beneficiaries of the partnership, should be kept informed.

Tuberculosis

Tuberculosis detection in private laboratories in the Syrian Arab Republic

- **Syrian Arab Republic**
  Nationwide
- **Study period**
  2006–2007

- **Small Grants Scheme**
  (SGS) 2006 No. 135

- **Principal Investigator**
  Fadia Maamari
  National Tuberculosis Control Programme
  Ministry of Health
  Damascus, Syrian Arab Republic
  e-mail: ntpsyria@mail.sy

Abstract

The aim of the study was to investigate the extent of private sector engagement in the diagnosis and management of tuberculosis (TB), and the extent of underreporting of sputum-smear-positive cases to the National Tuberculosis Control Programme (NTP). A comprehensive survey of all TB suspects referred to all private laboratories performing sputum-smear microscopy in the Syrian Arab Republic ($n = 285$) was conducted during the fourth quarter of 2007. Positive cases were traced back in the NTP registers to verify their status of registration at the NTP and evaluate the extent of underreporting of cases at the NTP.

Results During the fourth quarter of 2006, a total of 290 TB suspects were referred to private laboratories by private practitioners compared with 2041 referred to NTP laboratories. The reason for referral was to confirm diagnosis. Males constituted 72.2% of suspects, and 33% of suspects were aged between 25 and 34 years of age.

Of these suspects, 47 (12%) were sputum-smear positive, of which 41 were registered at the NTP and 6 were not. There was complete agreement between the diagnosis made in the NTP and in the private sector. Surveillance data showed that during the same quarter, 285 sputum-smear-positive cases were notified to the NTP.

Conclusion The NTP plays a major role in the diagnosis and treatment of TB cases in the country and only a limited proportion of cases are undetected by the NTP, suggesting a high case detection rate in the country.

Background

In 2006, the Syrian Arab Republic reported a treatment success rate of 89% but the case detection rate was only 48%. An in-depth review mission was carried out in 2006 to evaluate the programme performance regarding the different components of the Stop TB Strategy. Although several gaps in the case-finding process were identified, the mission concluded that the extent of underreporting of cases was less than 52% of cases in the country. This study aimed at investigating the extent of engagement of the private sector in the diagnosis and management of tuberculosis (TB), and the extent of underreporting of sputum-smear-positive cases to the National Tuberculosis Control Programme (NTP).

Materials and methods

A comprehensive survey of all TB suspects referred to all private laboratories performing sputum-smear microscopy in the country was conducted during the fourth quarter of 2007. Positive cases were traced back in the NTP registers to verify their status of registration at the NTP and evaluate the extent of underreporting of cases at the NTP.

Main study findings

A total of 290 TB suspects were referred to private laboratories during the study period. They consisted of 213 (73.2%) males and 77 (26.8%) females. Their age ranged from 15 to 80 years, and 287 (99%) were nationals. Sputum was the main specimen referred in 257 (89%) of suspects. Other specimens were bronchoalveolar lavage, urine, pleural fluid, spinal fluid and lymph nodes. Of

Conclusions and implications of the study

- The study reported that 87.2% of cases detected by private laboratories were referred or notified to the NTP. This is consistent with the 2006 surveillance data, which showed that around two thirds of patients were referred by private non-NTP providers (by referral of suspects or diagnosis and referral).
- These findings are consistent with the results of the in-depth review mission in 2006, which also confirmed that anti-TB drugs were only available at the NTP due to the ban of their selling in the private sector.
- This circumstantial evidence suggests that the case detection rate in the Syrian Arab Republic should be higher than the actually reported rates and that the estimated incidence of TB in the Syrian Arab Republic has been overestimated. Revisiting the Syrian Arab Republic estimated incidence is therefore recommended, based on this evidence.

these suspects, 47 (12%) were sputum-smear positive: 37 males and 10 females, and 2 were non-nationals. There was complete agreement between the diagnosis made in the NTP and in the private sector.

Regarding the status of registration of cases at the NTP, 41 (87.2%) of positive cases were found at the NTP registers, and only 6 were missing, of whom 2 were non-nationals.

Conclusions

The NTP plays a major role in the diagnosis and treatment of TB cases in the country and only a limited proportion of cases are undetected by the NTP. These results suggest a high TB case detection in the country and call for the need to revisit the Syrian Arab Republic estimated incidence.

Tuberculosis

Magnitude and determinants of non-compliance to treatment among pulmonary tuberculosis patients under DOTS in Lahore District, Pakistan

- **Pakistan**
  Punjab Province
- **Study period**
  July 2006–September 2007

- **Small Grants Scheme**
  (SGS) 2006 No. 70

- **Principal Investigator**
  Ayesha Humayun
  Centre for Health Research
  Fatima Memorial Hospital
  College of Medicine & Dentistry
  Lahore, Pakistan
  e-mail: drayeshah@gmail.com

Abstract

An ambidirectional study was conducted from July 2006 to September 2007 in Lahore District of the province of Punjab, Pakistan, to identify the extent of adherence of tuberculosis (TB) patients to anti-TB drug regimens and the factors that interfere with their successful completion of DOTS. A total of 421 new pulmonary TB patients who had started their treatment under DOTS during the study period were interviewed regarding the potential predictors/determinants of non-compliance and defaulting. These patients were reviewed at the end of the treatment period for treatment success and treatment interruption (default and non-compliance) was analysed in relation to the predictors.

Results At the end of the treatment period, 92.6% of patients had complied with their treatment and 7.3% had interrupted their treatment. Among the treatment interrupters, 25 (5.9% of all patients) were defaulters (treatment was interrupted for ≥ 2 months), while 6 (1.4% of all patients) were non-compliers (treatment was interrupted < 2 months).

Analysis showed a significantly increased risk of treatment interruption (both default and non-compliance) among: females (relative rate, RR: 2.08; 95% confidence interval, CI: 0.95–4.55); those who needed to travel in order to get medicine (RR: 20.78; 95% CI: 5.026–85.97; P < 0.0001); those who needed to travel a distance of more than 30 minutes' walk to get medicine (RR: 4.38; 95% CI: 2.22–8.63; *P* < 0.0001); those who sometimes needed to buy medicine (RR: 2.3; 95% CI: 1.173–4.51, *P* = 0.024); and those who were directly observed by a health-care provider (RR: 14.483; 95% CI: 4.95–42.374; *P* < 0.0001).

Conclusion Like sociodemographic, cultural and behavioural predictors of treatment interruption (default and non-compliance), DOTS was significantly associated with treatment compliance in TB high-burden countries. To improve treatment adherence and compliance, these factors should be addressed when reviewing strategies for TB control in Pakistan.

Background

Defaulting from tuberculosis (TB) treatment remains a major challenge for TB control programmes in the developing world. There is an increased risk of drug resistance, relapse, prolonged infectiousness and death among defaulters. The present study was conducted to determine the extent of treatment adherence (treatment interrupters and defaulters), and to identify the possible determining factors or predictors of treatment interruption.

Materials and methods

An ambidirectional study was conducted in Lahore District, the capital of Punjab Province, Pakistan. All new cases of pulmonary TB, who were resident in the district and were registered at any of the 32 diagnostic centres of the Punjab TB Control Programme in Lahore District during the period from 1 July 2006 to 31 January 2007 and who had started receiving DOTS therapy, were enrolled in the study.

Conclusions and implications of the study

- Female gender was a risk factor for non-compliance. This might be due to one of several reasons: the women had more responsibilities than men; their lack of authority in decision-making; or physical, psychological, domestic and cultural issues.
- Subjects who were observed by a health-care provider were at a higher risk of treatment interruption/default than those who were observed by a community or family member. The use of DOTS with free drug provision and the use of a home visitor should enhance compliance with treatment and hence cure of pulmonary TB.
- Community or family members are successful treatment supporters due to the fact that they belong to the same community and have the same socioeconomic and cultural background. Their counselling or advice will be more effective than that of a busy health-care provider as the patient needs emotional support, rather than plain advice, to swallow the bulk of tablets on a daily basis.

The study design combined elements of a prospective cohort study and a case–control study. A total of 421 eligible TB patients were traced in the district and then interviewed at home, regarding the determinants of non-compliance/defaulting. At the end of their treatment period, the cohort was categorized into compliers and treatment interrupters, the latter of which included non-compliers (treatment interruption <2 months) and defaulters (treatment interruption for ≥ 2 months). The frequency of treatment interruption (non-compliance and defaulters) was determined and compliers (controls) were compared with treatment interrupters (cases) regarding the predictors of non-compliance.

Main study findings

Of the 421 study participants, 177 (42.0%) were males and 244 (58.0%) were females; 390 (92.6%) of the participants had never stopped medicine and 31 (7.3%) had interrupted their treatment. Among these 31 subjects, 25 (80.6%) were defaulters (treatment interruption for ≥2 months), while 6 (19.4%) were non-compliers (treatment interruption for <2 months). The default rate was 5.9%.

Determinants of non-compliance

One hundred and seventy three (173; 41.1%) subjects had to get their medicine from DOTS treatment centres; among these patients only 6.4% had their own transport, while 26% walked and 67.6% used another mode of transportation to travel to the centres. Of these 173 patients, 105 (60.7%) travelled a distance further than 30 minutes' walk.

Gender-related factors were evaluated and the results showed that while 51.2% of females made the decision on their own to go to a treatment centre, 119 (48.8%) of females had to seek permission to go to a treatment centre; of these females 48.7% needed permission from their husband, 47.1 % from their parents and 4.2% from their in-laws.

A total of 43.9% of females expressed feelings of insecurity while travelling alone to the treatment centre, while 28.4% said seeking advice from a male doctor was difficult owing to cultural and religious reasons. Daily work load was also an issue for 51% of female subjects.

Evaluating knowledge, attitude and practice factors showed that 225 subjects (53.4%) felt stigmatized if anyone knew about their disease, 363 subjects (86.2%) had queries regarding side-effects of their anti-TB drugs, while 357 subjects (84.8%) had changed their diet due to TB. While 96.9% of subjects felt that they should continue and complete the course of treatment, 3.1% of subjects felt a false sense of cure after their initial intensive-phase treatment.

When asked whether they needed to buy anti-TB medicine on their own, 26.4% of subjects answered yes, but the majority (73.6%) of subjects said no. The majority of subjects (97.9%) said that their physician/health-care provider provided them with adequate information about pulmonary TB. When asked whether their physician/health-care provider instructed them about how to take medicine in terms of time, duration and method, the majority (98.1%) answered yes.

In 298 (70.8%) subjects, DOTS was carried out during the intensive phase of treatment but in 123 (29.2%) subjects DOTS was not done. In 16.1% of cases, a health-care provider was responsible for DOTS, while a family member or a person in the community was responsible for DOTS in 83.9% of subjects. On questioning about the nature of DOTS, 93.6% of subjects said they were observed until they swallowed the medicine.

The cure rate was confirmed using sputum-smear testing in 362 (86%) cases and found to be 91.7%.

The major reason for treatment interruption was lack of resources, especially financial ones. With regard to the time of treatment interruption, in 18 (58%) subjects, this occurred during the continuation phase of treatment.

Analysis showed a significantly increased risk of treatment interruption among: females; those who needed to travel to get medicine (odds ratio, OR: 24.77; 95% CI: 5.82–105.3); those who needed to travel a distance of more than 30 minutes' walk (OR: 5.12; 95% CI: 2.41–10.88); those who sometimes needed to buy medicine (OR: 2.48; 95% CI: 1.18–5.23); and those subjects who were directly observed by their health-care provider during the intensive phase of treatment (OR: 18.77; 95% CI: 5.90–59.67).

Conclusions and recommendations

This study reported a non-compliance rate of 7.3% among patients. The predictors of non-compliance or default were female sex, the need to travel for medicine, distance of the treatment centre from their home and the need to buy medicine. Patients' perceptions or the belief that there was no need to continue medicine after the intensive phase also made them at risk of being non-compliant or default. Direct observation by a responsible family member or neighbour was a protective factor against non-compliance or default.

Diagnosis

Egypt

Tuberculosis

Evaluation of different diagnostic techniques for improving sensitivity of direct microscopy for detection of acid-fast bacilli in sputum specimens in Alexandria, Egypt

- **Egypt**
  Alexandria Governorate
- **Study period**
  2005–2007

- **Small Grants Scheme**
  (SGS) 2005 No. 38

- **Principal Investigator**
  Safaa Amer
  Microbiology Department
  Faculty of Medicine
  Alexandria University, Egypt
  e-mail: dr_safaa_amer@yahoo.com

Abstract

The aim of the study was to evaluate the different sputum-processing techniques in improving sensitivity of direct microscopy for detection of acid-fast bacilli (AFB), thus improving the case detection rate as targeted by Egypt's National Tuberculosis Control Programme (NTCP). One thousand and two hundred (1200) sputum samples were collected from 600 patients with chest symptoms suggestive of tuberculosis (TB), who were attending four government chest clinics in Alexandria, Egypt (two specimens from each patient; first a spot specimen followed by an early morning specimen). Four Ziehl-Neelsen stained films were made from each specimen: direct smear, *N*-acetyl-L-cysteine (NALC) concentration technique, smear concentrated by cytocentrifugation (cytospin) and smear prepared by liquefaction of sputum with sodium hypochlorite (NaOCl) followed by concentration overnight. Sputum processed by NALC technique was then cultured on Lowenstein Jensen medium (to be used as a gold standard

Results Sensitivities of different microscopic techniques (spot and morning specimens, respectively) were as follow: direct (63.9, 60.9), NALC (73.6, 67.6), cytospin (83.3, 77) and NaOCl (66.7, 64.9). Thus cytospin technique showed the highest sensitivity and highest percentage of accuracy (98.97%), followed by NALC (97.96%) and, finally, NaOCl and direct smear which gave the lowest accuracy. Smears prepared by processing by different concentration techniques showed an increased rate of detection of AFB when compared by direct microscopy. Again, cytospin technique was the only technique that gave a statistically significant increase in rate of detection (17.8% increase). All microscopic techniques were 100% specific.

Conclusion Processing of sputum by various chemicals and centrifugation or overnight precipitation increased sensitivity of microscopic detection of AFB compared with direct smear. Cytospin technique gave the highest sensitivity, accuracy and significant rate of detection of AFB.

Background

Early identification and isolation of tuberculosis (TB) patients is of utmost importance in minimizing the risk of further epidemic spread. Smear microscopy is currently the most feasible microbiological method for initial diagnosis of pulmonary TB in developing countries, where 95% of TB cases and 98% of deaths occur. Although this conventional technique of direct smear examination with Ziehl-Neelsen staining is cheap and easy to perform, its low sensitivity is a major drawback.

The gold standard method for definitive diagnosis of TB is by the clinical laboratory growth on culture of *Mycobacterium tuberculosis* from patient specimens. However, these slow-growing organisms have a generation time of up to 22 h. Thus, it could take 4–8 weeks for a positive culture.

Deficiencies in current case-finding tools in disease-endemic countries have made it difficult to ensure access to good diagnostics at all health-service levels, leaving many patients undiagnosed. New cost-effective alternative techniques are urgently needed in Egypt. Improvements in the sensitivity of smear microscopy would allow earlier diagnosis. TB programmes could then optimize disease control from a public-health standpoint, as well as improve individual patient management. Recently, different workers reported that the concentration of sputum by sedimentation, with or without cytocentrifugation, resulted in increased detection of mycobacteria in clinical specimens.

The aim of this study was to evaluate the diagnostic validity of different sputum-processing techniques in detection of acid-fast bacilli (AFB) in sputum, as compared to the conventional technique of direct smear examination with Ziehl-Neelsen staining.

Conclusions and implications of the study

- Cytospin technique increased the sensitivity of sputum-smear microscopy by 17.5% compared with the direct smear method (80% versus 62.5%, respectively), and showed a high agreement with culture. The technique proved to be a simple, rapid and safe diagnostic tool for TB.
- It is recommended that this tool for routine diagnosis of TB is introduced into NTCP TB management units.

Materials and methods

The study was carried out at four government chest clinics in Alexandria, Egypt (Ministry of Health and Population DOTS facilities) namely: Maamoura, Moharrem Bey, Gomrok and Kom El-shokafa. Two sputum specimens (first a spot specimen followed by an early morning one) were collected in sterile disposable plastic cups from 600 new patients with suspected pulmonary TB.

Each sputum specimen was processed by four methods for microscopic examination: the direct method; the *N*-acetyl-L-cysteine (NALC) concentration method with 2% sodium hydroxide (NaOH); sputum smears concentrated by cytocentrifugation technique; and liquefaction of sputum with sodium hypochlorite (NaOCl) followed by concentration of bacilli through overnight sedimentation.

Regarding culture, examination was first carried out within 72 h after inoculation to detect contaminants; thereafter, cultures were examined weekly: after 1 week to detect rapidly growing mycobacteria, and after 3–8 weeks to detect cultures of *Mycobacterium tuberculosis* as well as other slow-growing mycobacteria.

Main study findings

One thousand and two hundred (1200) sputum specimens (600 spot specimens and 600 morning specimens) were examined for AFB by direct smears, and smears after concentration by: NALC, cytocentrifugation and sedimentation overnight with NaOCl. Out of 600 spot sputum specimens, 7.6% were positive by direct smear, 8.8% were positive by NALC, 10% were positive by cytocentrifugation, 8% by NaOCl and 12% by culture. The corresponding rates for the 600 morning sputum specimens were 7.5%, 8.3%, 9.5%, 8% and 12.3%, respectively. Although the rates of detection of AFB were slightly higher by different microscopic techniques in spot specimens than in morning specimens, the differences were not statistically significant. On the other hand, rate of detection by culture was higher in morning specimens than in spot specimens, but again the difference was not statistically significant.

By direct smear, 46 spot and 45 morning specimens were true positive, giving a sensitivity of 64% and 61%, respectively. For the NALC method, 53 spot and 50 morning specimens were true positive, giving sensitivities of 74% and 68%, respectively. As regards the cytospin method, 60 spot and 57 morning specimens were true positive, giving and sensitivities of 83% and 77%, respectively. For the NaOCl method, 48 spot and 48 morning specimens were true positive, giving sensitivities of 67% and 65%, respectively. All microscopic methods were 100% specific as there were no false-positive cases detected by any method.

Results of cytospin technique when compared with culture results showed the highest percentage of accuracy (98% and 97% in spot and morning specimens) followed by NALC (97% and 96% in spot and morning specimens) and finally NaOCl and direct-smear techniques, which gave nearly the same percentage of accuracy.

Again using the Kappa test, cytospin technique showed the highest agreement with culture results (very good agreement; 0.898 and 0.855) followed by NALC technique (very good agreement; 0.831 and 0.785), then NaOCl technique (good agreement; 0.779 and 0.764) and finally direct smear (good agreement; 0.757, 0.731).

Processing of sputum by cytospin technique produced an increase of smear sensitivity of 17.5% when compared with direct smear (62.5% by direct smear versus 80% by cytospin technique). For NALC technique, the increase in mean sensitivity was 8.5% (62.5% by direct smear versus 71% by NALC technique). NaOCl technique showed a 3.5% increase in mean sensitivity (62.5% by direct smear versus 66% by NaOCl technique). However, the increase of rate of detection of positive specimens when direct smear results were compared with other processing techniques was only statistically significant for cytospin technique (two-tailed P value = 0.0012)

Conclusions and recommendations

Processing of sputum by various chemicals and centrifugation or overnight precipitation increased sensitivity of microscopic detection of AFB compared with direct smear. Cytospin technique gave the highest sensitivity, accuracy and significant rate of detection of AFB. Added to that, it is rapid, safe, cost effective and simple for rapid diagnosis of TB in the NTCP. Sputum processing by NaOCl technique followed by overnight precipitation was on average more sensitive than direct microscopy with clearer field and high bacillus concentration, which made this technique appropriate for diagnostic centres not equipped with a cytocentrifuge.

Tuberculosis

Evaluating DOTS compliance in an urban area of Tehran based on the health belief model

- **Islamic Republic of Iran**
  Tehran
- **Study period**
  2002–2006

- **Small Grants Scheme**
  (SGS) 2005 No. 116

- **Principal Investigator**
  Rahim Taghizadeh Asl
  National Research Institute of Tuberculosis and Lung Disease (NRITLD)
  Shahid Beheshti University of Medical Sciences
  Tehran, Islamic Republic of Iran
  e-mail: taghizadehasl@yahoo.com

Abstract

A cross-sectional study was carried out during 2005–2006 whereby all newly registered tuberculosis (TB) patients at the National Research Institute of Tuberculosis and Lung Disease (NRITLD) and four urban health centres in Tehran were recruited for the study. A questionnaire was used to assess the determinants of patients' compliance with DOTS and also their perceptions using different components of the health belief model (HBM). The association between the components of the HBM with compliance was tested using principle component analysis for data reduction and the *t* test or its non-parametric equivalent test.

Results Of 152 enrolled consented patients, 57 (37.5%) were compliant with DOTS. A total of 57% of patients had received some education about TB during the course of their treatment. There was no difference in education between compliant and non-compliant cases. Comparing the mean scores of different components of the HBM showed that the perceived severity and perceived benefit were significantly higher in the compliant, compared with the non-compliant, groups. There was no significant difference between the two groups regarding the preferred methods of education.

Conclusion The study showed that compliance to treatment under direct supervision is still poor in the Islamic Republic of Iran. In order to increase DOTS compliance, it is important to emphasize the health education of patients during the course of treatment, stressing the benefits of proper treatment and the severity of the disease and drug resistance in the case of non-adherence to treatment.

Background

The national tuberculosis (TB) programme was initiated in 1995 in the Islamic Republic of Iran and reported 100% coverage of DOTS. However, there was a gap in implementing DOTS in urban areas. The aim of this study was to determine the factors related to compliance with DOTS among TB patients using the health belief model (HBM). The HBM states that the perception of a personal health behaviour threat is itself influenced by at least three factors: general health values, which include interest and concern about health; specific health beliefs about vulnerability to a particular health threat; and beliefs about the consequences of the health problem. Once an individual perceives a threat to their health and is simultaneously cued to action, and if their perceived benefits outweigh their perceived threats, then that individual is most likely to undertake the recommended preventive health action [1].

Materials and methods

In order to design the questionnaire, a qualitative study (a grounded theory design) was first carried out through focus-group discussions and in-depth interviews with a number of patients and TB experts working at local and national levels of the Iranian TB surveillance system. The results of this study were then used to design a quantitative questionnaire. This preparation for the first draft of the questionnaire took about 2 month. A self-administered quantitative questionnaire was then prepared for the assessment of knowledge, attitude and

Conclusions and implications of the study

- Compliance with DOTS was reported in only 37.5% of patients in urban Tehran. Compliance was not affected by age, sex, or the patient's preferred source of health education. The preferred source of health education is the treating physician.
- The HBM showed that the perceived severity and perceived benefit were significantly higher in the compliant compared to the non-compliant group.
- The concept of DOTS is acceptable for patients but there is a lack of organization and information about DOTS to patients. More emphasis on the health education of patients during the course of treatment is recommended. This should stress the benefits of proper treatment and the severity of the disease in case of non-adherence to therapy.

behaviour of patients regarding DOTS and TB treatment, considering main components of the HBM. Before use, the designed questionnaire was tested for its validity and reliability.

A cross-sectional study was carried out during 2005–2006 whereby all new registered TB patients in the National Institute of Tuberculosis and Lung Disease (NRITLD) and four urban health centres in Tehran were recruited for the study. Each case was interviewed using the pretested and structured questionnaire, which collected information about the time of onset of the symptoms of his/her illness, time of diagnosis of the current disease, adherence to DOTS protocol, demographic data etc. Also health staff in health centres of Shahid Beheshti University and specialists in the NRITLD were interviewed about DOTS and obstacles to compliance.

The questionnaire was designed to address the following components of the HBM [1]:

- Perceived susceptibility. Each individual has his/her own perception of the likelihood of experiencing a condition that would adversely affect their health.
- Perceived seriousness. This refers to the beliefs that a person holds concerning the effect that a given disease or condition would have on their state of affairs.
- Perceived benefits of taking action. Taking action towards prevention of a disease or dealing with an illness is the next step to expect after an individual has accepted their susceptibility to a disease and recognized its seriousness. The direction of action that a person chooses will be influenced by their beliefs regarding this action.
- Barriers to taking action. Barriers to taking action relate to the characteristics of a treatment or preventive measure, for example it may be inconvenient, expensive, unpleasant, painful or upsetting. These characteristics may lead a person away from taking the desired action.
- Cues to action. An individual's perception of the levels of susceptibility and seriousness provide the force to act. Benefits (minus barriers) provide the path of action.

Non-compliant cases were defined as TB cases who had not taken their drugs under direct observation.

To implement the quantitative parts of the study and design the questionnaire, we began by investigating feasible methods of data gathering and also our access to patients under treatment in hospital and in public health services.

All of the notified cases in the NRITLD were initially registered in a project and history file. The cases under treatment were interviewed when they came to follow-up treatment. There was a physician in each centre who was directly involved with cases during treatment and he/she filled out the questionnaire at each follow-up visit for treatment. Self-administered questionnaires were given to the patient and filed.

TB cases registered over a 5-month period were enrolled. Compliance was recorded at the time of routine follow-up by the responsible physicians in the the 5th month. New cases in the following months were added to the list by the district TB coordinator.

However, at the NRITLD there were two different types of TB cases. The first group were inpatients during the first weeks or month of treatment, while the second group had taken drugs as outpatients.

Diagnosed cases were also enrolled from hospital files and types of disease and cases were categorized. To extract new TB cases who arrived after the start of the project, it was necessary to locate both inpatient and outpatient cases, which was very time-consuming, but mandatory to achieving maximum size of diagnosed TB cases in hospital.

Main study findings

The qualitative survey

The majority of the interviewed patients in the focus-group discussions had been treated for more than 2 months (and mostly for about 5 months). Most of these patients believed that they had caught TB from dust in the air and most had been ill for about 3 weeks to 6 months before diagnosis. They had also attended many physicians before a definite diagnosis of TB was made. Most patients believed that TB carried a social stigma and preferred not to be identified as a TB patient in their community, job or even among family and friends. Most patients believed that they had got better since the start of treatment. However, some mentioned that lay people did not accept that a TB patient could be cured with proper treatment for the rest of their life. All patients agreed that they needed more information about TB and that this was also true for the general community. Most thought that TV and radio were the best ways for teaching the community about TB.

Most patients thought it was very important to be properly trained in the use of drugs and to be aware of possible adverse reactions and said that they would have benefited from such knowledge. Many patients preferred to get drugs and follow-up services from a health centre located near their home. Some patients had problems affording the laboratory and radiology costs, while many said that they had not paid for drugs during the course of their treatment.

Most patients thought that some support was needed to maintain their treatment during the 6-month period, and especially during the first 2 months of treatment. However, they believed daily direct observation was not required for ordinary patients, since it might result in reducing patients' confidence in their treatment. However, they thought daily observation of treatment by another person should be used for handicapped patients and children. Some patients mentioned they did not like to be observed by others when taking their drugs, especially by someone who was neither a family member nor health worker. Almost all of the patients complained about the great quantity of pills they had to take during the course of treatment, as well as the treatment's long duration. This was especially troublesome during the first 2 months of treatment. A number of patients mentioned that they suffered from at least one adverse effect from their anti-TB drugs during the course of their treatment but none mentioned giving up treatment because of this.

In-depth interviews with specialists

According to the results of these in-depth interviews, most patients know something about TB but their knowledge is not sufficient to change wrong attitudes. There are some problems with diagnosing TB. One problem results from patients being afraid of TB, denying their symptoms and postponing an examination for diagnosis and the follow-up of their disease. Another problem is that diagnosis is delayed as TB often does not appear in a doctor's differential diagnosis. A further problem is the lack of skilled personnel in laboratories for diagnosing TB. There is also a lack of communication between private and government sectors, and some problems in recording and reporting patients from the private sector and health-care systems, other than those directly under the supervision of the Ministry of Health.

Quantitative results

Most TB patients were non-compliant with DOTS; of 152 enrolled consented patients, only 57 (37.5%) were compliant with DOTS. A total of 57% of patients had received some education about TB during the course of their care and treatment. The majority of patient preferred doctors to be the primary source of their health education during their TB treatment. The secondary source of health education was TV.

The study was performed in the largest city of the Islamic Republic of Iran, thus the results may not be generalizable to other parts of the country such as small towns, where to general practitioners may be better. However, DOTS access performance is an important issue in large cities. There was no significant difference between compliant and non-compliant groups regarding age, sex, or type of preferred source of health educations, with both groups preferring their treating physicians.

On the other hand, there was a significant association between severity and benefit components of the HBM and compliance with DOTS. According to the questionnaire, most of the severity questions showed the fear of patients with regard to stigmatization. Most patients liked to be supervised by another person. Most patients were ashamed of TB, perceiving it as a bad and evil disease.

Conclusions and recommendations

Compliance to DOTS is still poor in the Islamic Rebublic of Iran. In order to increase DOTS compliance, it is important to place emphasis on the health education of patients during the course of their treatment, stressing the benefits of proper treatment and the severity of the disease in case of non-adherence to therapy. It is important to understand that the preferred source of health education is the treating physician, who should spend more time talking to and educating their patients.

References

[1] DeBarr KA. A review of current health education theories. *Californian Journal of Health Promotion*, 2004, 2:74–87.

Vaccine-preventable diseases

Susceptibility to rubella in pregnant women and to measles in high-risk groups in the Syrian Arab Republic

- **Syrian Arab Republic**
  Damascus, Rural Damascus, Aleppo, Hama, Lattakia and Hasakah governorates
- **Study period**
  2006–2007
- **Small Grants Scheme**
  (SGS) 2006 No. 5

- **Principal Investigator**
  Haifa Nasri
  Vaccine Preventable Disease Programme
  Ministry of Health
  Damascus, Syrian Arab Republic

Abstract

A study was conducted to investigate rubella susceptibility in pregnant women and measles susceptibility among high-risk groups in the Syrian Arab Republic and to identify some risk factors associated with susceptibility. After obtaining an informed consent, blood samples were obtained from 968 pregnant women attending health-care centres for antenatal care. The serum was tested for rubella immunoglobulin G (IgG) using enzyme-linked immunosorbent assay (ELISA). Blood samples were also obtained from 1365 children from three minority groups (gypsies, Bedouins and non-nationals, mainly Iraqis), after obtaining an informed consent, and the serum was tested for measles IgG using ELISA.

Results The overall proportion of susceptible, rubella-IgG seronegative pregnant females was 4.0%. The highest proportion of susceptible females was in Lattakia (10.6%) compared with Damascus, where only 1.2% of the pregnant women were susceptible. There was no significant difference in prevalence between urban and rural areas. Susceptibility decreased with age to reach 0% at 40 years and was inversely proportional to the number of pregnancies and abortions, and significantly lower in those with a history of a newborn with congenital rubella syndrome (CRS) or a history of febrile rash illness during pregnancy.

Overall, 8.9% of subjects from the minority groups lacked antibodies to measles. The proportions of susceptible individuals were 10.4%, 8.6 and 7.6% among Bedouins, Iraqis and gypsies, respectively. By age group, susceptibility was 12.3% among children in the 2–5 year age group, 7% in the 5–8 year age group and 8.5 % in the 8–15 year age group.

Overall, almost 90% of the 1365 participants reported receiving their routine measles vaccine. Reported measles vaccine coverage was 98.7% among Iraqis, 90.3% among Bedouins and 64.4% among gypsies. The distribution according to age groups was: 88% among 2–5 years, 90% among 5–8 years and 83.7 among 8–15 years. Overall, 88.5% of Bedouins, 52% of gypsies and 3.9% of Iraqis had been covered by routine immunization through mobile teams.

Conclusion The study reported a low rate of susceptibility to rubella in pregnant women in the Syrian Arab Republic. However, a high susceptibility for measles was reported among high-risk groups.

Background

Rubella is a mild viral disease. However, the virus can cross the placenta, causing serious consequences. Fetal death, miscarriages, stillbirths and congenital rubella syndrome (CRS) may occur as a result of intrauterine infection,

Conclusions and implications of the study

- The proportion of immune, seropositive, pregnant women in the Syrian Arab Republic was 96%, which is high enough to halt the indigenous transmission of rubella virus. However, the highest proportion of susceptible females was in the age range 18–35 years and in order to protect future mothers and their fetuses maintain a high level of immunity in this age group vaccination campaigns aimed at young girls and unmarried females who are younger than 35 years of age should be considered.
- The study reported a moderate measles susceptibility rate. However, the rate increased to 12.3% in the 2–5 year age group, and to 10.4% among Bedouins, and there was low coverage (49% among age group 2–6 years), despite the previous measles follow-up campaign. In order to achieve the elimination target of maintaining 95% immunity to measles in each cohort in every district, the following are recommended:
  - implementing a house-to-house mopping-up campaign among these high-risk groups, using MMR vaccine to cover the age group from 9 months to 15 years;
  - determining the most suitable means of covering these groups on a regular basis;
  - implementing yearly measles campaign supplementary immunization activities to cover these groups.

particularly during the first trimester of pregnancy. CRS can lead to many birth defects, including deafness, heart disease and cataracts; this is the main reason a vaccine for rubella was developed. The combined vaccine measles, mumps and rubella (MMR) is recommended at 12–15 months, with a second dose when the child is 4–6 years old. Rubella vaccination is particularly important for non-immune women who may become pregnant, because of the risk of serious birth defects if they acquire the disease during pregnancy. Therefore, it is essential to consider vaccination of all women of childbearing age in any rubella-control strategy.

The Syrian Arab Republic has achieved a high measles coverage rate of up to 98% in recent years. However, measles outbreaks still occur, jeopardizing efforts towards measles elimination. Observations suggest these outbreaks could be attributed to low coverage rates in high-risk groups, including gypsies, Bedouins and non-nationals, mainly Iraqis. The population of the first two groups is estimated to be around 300 000, compared with 1.3 million Iraqis within a total Syrian population of 19.2 million. In order to control sporadic outbreaks, attention needs to be given to these minority groups. Surveying these groups to determine their immune status against measles will help further planning to control measles throughout the country. A study was therefore conducted to investigate rubella susceptibility in pregnant women and measles susceptibility among high-risk groups in the Syrian Arab Republic and to identify some of the risk factors associated with susceptibility.

Materials and methods

A cross-sectional descriptive study was conducted whereby the country was divided into six geographic regions (Damascus, Rural Damascus, Aleppo, Hama, Lattakia and Hasakah. governorates) and the clustering technique was used on two levels: districts and health centres. During the months of August and September, 2006, a total of 968 pregnant women attending randomly selected primary health-care centres for antenatal care in the Syrian Arab Republic were consecutively enrolled until the estimated sample size allocated to each centre was completed. Those who consented were asked to complete a detailed questionnaire, which included questions on sociodemographic characteristics, risk factors, history of exposure to rubella during pregnancy, rubella immunization and knowledge about rubella. The pregnant women were also asked to give a blood sample for detection of immunoglobulin G (IgG) antibodies to rubella virus in serum, using the quantitative enzyme-linked immunosorbent assay (ELISA).

To study measles susceptibility among high-risk groups, a cross-sectional survey was conducted whereby 1365 children between 2 and 15 years were randomly selected from three minority groups: 432 gypsies, 481 Bedouins and 452 Iraq distributed in seven governorates. A specially designed questionnaire was used to collect information covering sociodemographic characteristics, vaccination coverage (self-reported and cards), history of measles, reasons for non-vaccination, mobile team coverage, knowledge/attitudes regarding vaccination, and predictors of non-vaccination. Sera collected from these children were tested for measles IgG using ELISA.

Main study findings

Of a total of 968 consenting pregnant women, 928 (95.9%) were rubella seropositive, 39 (4%) were seronegative and 1 had an equivocal result. Women aged 18–35 years were the most susceptible ($P = 0.048$). Susceptibility was inversely proportional to the number of pregnancies and abortions, and was significantly lower among those with a history of previous fetal death, history of a newborn suffering from CRS or a history of febrile rash illness during pregnancy.

Of a total number of 1365 consenting individuals from the high-risk groups, 85.9% were measles IgG positive, 5.1% had equivocal results and 8.9% were measles IgG negative. Measles susceptibility rate was highest (12.3%) among the 2–5 years age group, despite the national follow-up campaign that directly preceded this survey and included this age group. Also, susceptibility rates to measles virus were highest (10.4%) among Bedouins, which may be the result of the low routine coverage among this group in some areas.

Conclusions

The study reported a low rate of susceptibility to rubella in pregnant women in the Syrian Arab Republic. However, the highest proportion of susceptible females was in the age range 18–35 years and so in order to protect future mothers and their fetuses, vaccination campaigns aimed at young girls and unmarried females younger than 35 years of age should be considered.

A high susceptibility to measles among high-risk groups was also reported, highlighting the need to carry out mopping-up campaigns and strengthen the routine immunization among these high-risk groups to achieve the elimination target.

Pakistan

Vaccine-peventable diseases

Increasing tetanus toxoid coverage of women of childbearing age through behaviour change communication in Lahore district, Pakistan

- **Pakistan**
  Lahore district, Punjab Province
- **Study period**
  2005–2006
- **Small Grants Scheme**
  (SGS) 2005 No. 153

- **Principal Investigator**
  Tayyaba Nasreen
  Save The Mother Fund Society (SMFS)
  Lahore, Pakistan
  e-mail: tnasreen_smfs@yahoo.com

Abstract

A study was carried out in Punjab Province, Pakistan, with the objective of increasing the tetanus toxoid (TT) coverage among women of childbearing age (CBAs) and increasing awareness of the importance of TT vaccination among those women, their husbands and other family members who may affect decision-making about getting TT vaccination. The study evaluated the use of behaviour change communication (BCC) strategy in increasing TT coverage among CBAs and was conducted in rural union council UC147 of Lahore district, Punjab Province, which has a population of almost 50 000, scattered among 10 villages. Punjab is the most populous province in Pakistan, with a population of 80.3 million in an area of 205 345 km^2. A baseline survey was completed before starting the interventions and a postintervention survey was conducted in September 2006.

Results The majority of the respondents (86%) had heard about the TT vaccination. A substantial number of husbands said that they had not heard about this vaccination previously. The "vaccinator" was the prime source of information for the majority of the respondents (47%), followed by information from relatives and friends (19%), then TV and radio (9.5%). Despite the very high rates of deliveries in rural areas by traditional birth attendants (TBAs), their role in spreading information about TT vaccination was almost negligible (0.3%); similarly, very few people gave lady health workers (LHWs) as the prime source of TT vaccination information. A large number of respondents (30%), including CBAs and mothers-in-law, said that TT vaccination was good only for the child's health. More than one fifth of the participants (mostly husbands and fathers-in-law) had no idea about the benefits of TT vaccination.

After the intervention, considerable improvement was seen in the knowledge base of the community during the focus group discussions (FGDs) and individual interviews. There was also a considerable increase in the number of women opting for further doses of TT vaccination and in recordkeeping.

The intervention was able to change the prevalent practice of giving less attention to mothers' health through community mobilization in the form of meetings with large groups. The impact of these gatherings was increased due to continuity of word of mouth generated from these meetings. During the intervention, the health service providers, especially LHWs, played an important role in bringing about a positive change and resulting in their own role being magnified in the community. They are now respected as life-saver agents, rather than purely family-planning advisers.

Conclusion Continuity of community orientation sessions is recommended to ensure sustained behavioural modification and practice. The visiting schedule of vaccinators should be improved and should target communities and availability of vaccination should be ensured. Linking the polio vaccination campaigns with TT vaccination campaigns is recommended.

Background

Tetanus is a vaccine-preventable disease that causes an annual total of 309 000 deaths. Of particular concern is maternal and neonatal tetanus (MNT), which represents a triple failure of public health in terms of routine vaccinations, antenatal care and clean delivery/umbilical-cord care services. MNT is a swift and painful killer that killed about 200 000 newborns in 2000. The goal of MNT elimination was declared jointly

Conclusions and implications of the study

- There is a need to raise awareness about symptoms, causes and communicability of tetanus.
- There is also a need for better training for health workers, including LHWs, TBAs and doctors, to ensure better treatment of patients.
- Community health-education sessions should be continued to ensure sustained behaviour modification and practice.
- Visiting schedules of vaccinators to target communities should be improved and availability of vaccination should be ensured.
- Linking polio vaccination campaigns with TT vaccination campaigns is recommended.

by the United Nations Children's Fund (UNICEF), WHO and the United Nations Population Fund (UNFPA), with the establishment of a global fund for MNT elimination.

The three key strategies for achieving MNT elimination recommended by WHO/UNICEF/UNFPA are: provision of at least two doses of tetanus toxoid (TT2) to all pregnant women in high-risk areas and three doses (TT3) to all women of childbearing age (CBAs); promotion of clean delivery services to all pregnant women; and ensuring effective surveillance for MNT. There is a renewed momentum to achieve MNT elimination in the 57 countries that have not yet done so. However, 90% of the neonatal deaths occur in 27 of the 57 countries. Pakistan is one of the eight high-burden countries that account for about 73% of neonatal tetanus deaths.

In Pakistan, 50% of districts are at high risk for MNT. In a study conducted in Peshawar district, North West Frontier Province, Pakistan, 65% of women in urban areas were vaccinated, while in rural areas 60% were vaccinated. Females in the urban areas were older and had more knowledge regarding TT vaccination than females in the rural areas. More women in the urban areas had made antenatal care visits (79%) than those in rural areas (50%).

There are extremely wide variations in TT vaccination coverage from district to district. In 2004, it was estimated that TT vaccination coverage for all districts of Punjab was as follows: one dose of TT (TT1), 49%; two doses (TT2), 37%; and three, four and five doses (TT3, TT4 and TT5) were from 5% to 10%.

Behaviour change communication (BCC) is a multilevel tool for promoting and sustaining risk-reducing behaviour change in individuals and communities by distributing tailored health messages using a variety of communication channels.

Materials and methods

This study was a mixture of quantitative and qualitative research. The study was implemented in one rural union council of Lahore district, UC147, which has a population of about 50 000 located in 10 villages with three basic health units. The target union council is situated south of Lahore, the provincial capital city.

This was a quasi-experimental (pre- and postintervention) study design and data for the baseline/end-line surveys were collected using structured questionnaires. In the quantitative survey, 20 households were selected from each village (a total of 200 from 10 villages) and in each household all the eligible respondents, 300 in total, were interviewed before and after the intervention. Four different questionnaires, one for each type of respondent, were developed as follows: for married women of childbearing age (CBAs), including pregnant women (15–49 years of age); for mothers-in-law of married CBAs; for husbands of married CBAs; and for fathers-in-law of married CBAs. Before finalizing these instruments, they were pretested in a non-intervention area.

The baseline survey was completed before starting the interventions to collect information on concepts, views and apprehensions held by participants about tetanus and its vaccination. Information was collected from the respondents (300 in the pre- and post-intervention) regarding knowledge about tetanus, including its mode of infection, seriousness, signs and symptoms; knowledge about malpractices during delivery that may contribute to tetanus development; knowledge about TT vaccination method, and advantages and disadvantages of vaccination; TT vaccination status and reasons for not getting TT vaccine, if not vaccinated (from married CBAs only); and suggestions to improve TT coverage.

In addition to individual interviews, five focus-group discussions (FGDs) were conducted by social scientists in five villages, before and after the intervention. The FGDs were for: married CBAs, including pregnant women (15–49 years of age); mothers-in-law of married CBAs; husbands of married CBAs; fathers-in-law of married CBAs; and traditional birth attendants (TBAs), lady health workers (LHWs) and vaccinators.

An end-line survey was conducted in September 2006 to measure the change in knowledge about vaccination and TT coverage among CBAs following the implementation of the BCC strategy. The same methodology was used as for the baseline survey.

Training-of-trainer workshop

Health-management committee members (536 persons) attended 20 training-of-trainer workshops (10 for females, 10 for males) conducted in 10 villages of the project area. The committee members were trained to conduct health-awareness programmes at community level. Their goal was to persuade reluctant families to get married CBAs vaccinated. Trainees were given information, education and communication materials covering: mother and child health care; reasons women may die during pregnancy or labour; danger signs in pregnancy, delivery and postdelivery in women and in newborn babies; and TT vaccination and neonatal tetanus. The trained committee members and LHWs then conducted 54 health education programmes in their communities to increase knowledge among the targeted population about health issues and TT vaccination.

Main study findings

Baseline survey

The majority of the respondents (77.1%) were illiterate/uneducated; only 10.7% of respondents had primary-level qualifications. Almost all mothers-in-law and fathers-in-law were illiterate. Although the majority of the respondents (86%) had heard about TT vaccination, a substantial number of husbands said that they had not heard about this vaccination. The "vaccinator" was the prime source of information for the majority of the respondents (47%), followed by information from relatives and friends (19%), and TV and radio (9.5%). Despite the very high percentage of deliveries in rural areas conducted by TBAs, their role in spreading information about TT vaccination was almost negligible (0.3%). Similarly, very few people cited LHWs as their prime source of TT vaccination information.

A total of 30% of all respondents, including CBAs and mothers-in-law, thought that TT vaccination was only good for the child's health and more than 20% of all participants (mostly husbands and fathers-in-law) had no knowledge about the benefits of TT vaccination. A total of 30% of all respondents cited lack of knowledge about the importance of TT vaccination as the main reason for not getting vaccinated, while 5% cited non-belief in vaccination mainly on religious grounds as their reason for not getting TT vaccination.

FGDs

In the FGDs, knowledge about tetanus was very poor in women and TBAs, and virtually non-existent in males. Apart from LHWs and vaccinators, no one had any proper information about the seriousness, signs/symptoms and dangers associated with non-vaccinated women. Although the rate of vaccination of pregnant women was increasing, this was mainly to save the life of the child and not of the mother. No proper schedule, record-keeping and follow-up programmes were in operation.

End-line survey

Considerable improvement in the knowledge base of the community was shown during the postintervention individual interviews and FGDs, indicating that the BCC interventions played an important role in eradicating ill-conceived deterrents to TT vaccination. There was also a considerable increase in the number of women opting for further doses of TT vaccination and in keeping records. Community meetings with large groups helped to change the prevalent practice of giving less attention to mothers' health. The impact of these meetings was increased through subsequent word-of-mouth communication generated by these meetings.

During the intervention the health-service providers, especially the LHWs, played an important role in bringing about positive change, resulting in their role in the community being improved. They are now respected as life-savers, rather than just family-planning advisors.

Conclusions and recommendations

Continuity of community orientation sessions is recommended to ensure sustained behavioural modification and practice. The visiting schedule of vaccinators should be improved and should target communities and availability of vaccination should be ensured. Linking the polio vaccination campaigns with TT vaccination campaigns is recommended.

Vaccine-preventable diseases

Immunogenicity and efficacy of the Hoshino strain of mumps (included in MMR vaccine) against mumps in Shahr-e-kord, Islamic Republic of Iran

- **Islamic Republic of Iran**
  Shahr-e-kord District
- **Study period**
  December 2004–December 2006
- **Small Grants Scheme**
  (SGS) 2006 No. 100

- **Principal Investigator**
  Majid Avijgan
  AlZahra Hospital,
  Shahr-e-kord
  Islamic Republic of Iran
  e-mail: avijgan@yahoo.com

Abstract

The report describes the immunogenicity of the Hoshino strain of mumps, included in the mumps, measles and rubella (MMR) vaccine, in Shahr-e-kord, Islamic Republic of Iran. A total of 338 children aged 3–18 years were tested for mumps immunoglobulin G (IgG) using enzyme-linked immunosorbent assay (ELISA).

Results The proportion of susceptible, mumps IgG-negative children was 19.8% (67 subjects). Of the 67 susceptible children, 36 received the MMR vaccination and successfully completed the study. Blood was collected by venipuncture 3, 12 and 24 months after vaccination and serum samples were tested by ELISA for detection of mumps immunoglobulin M (IgM) and IgG. The overall seroconversion rate was 86.1%, 77.7% and 75% at 3, 12 and 24 months, respectively.

Conclusion The study reported that 86.1% of subjects became immune to mumps following one dose of MMR vaccine. This rate indicates that there is about 14% vaccine failure. A steady decline in the proportion of immune children was observed when tested at 3, 12 and 24 months after receiving the vaccine. The proportion of immune children 24 months following immunization was 75%, and 25% of the children tested remained non-immune and susceptible.

Background

As in many other developing countries, mumps remains one of the causes of morbidity among children in the Islamic Republic of Iran. In March 2004, mumps immunization was integrated into the expanded programme of immunization and combined with measles and rubella (mumps, measles and rubella, MMR). However, no data on the community herd immunity against mumps or persistency of antibodies against the Hoshino strain of mumps (included in the MMR vaccine) were available before this integration. This study was conducted to evaluate the immunogenicity, efficacy and long-term immunity of the Hoshino strain of mumps (included in the MMR vaccine) against mumps in Shahr-e-kord, Islamic Republic of Iran, 2 years after MMR vaccination in a group of seronegative susceptible children.

Materials and methods

Over a 24-month period from December 2004 to December 2006, children aged 3–18 years old were selected from 158 schools and 100 day-care centres by the stratified random sampling method. The size of the sample in each stratum was taken in proportion to the size of the stratum. A sample size of 338 children aged 3–18 years old was selected (56.5% boys).

A well-designed questionnaire was used by the interviewers to collect sociodemographic data. After obtaining informed consent from the parents, a 10-ml blood sample was withdrawn from each participant. Blood specimens were collected on the day of vaccination, then at 3, 12 and 24 months postvaccination. Blood specimens were centrifuged and sera were stored in cryovials at -20 °C until all samples were tested simultaneously

Conclusions and implications of the study

- Although 86% of children were seroconverted immediately postvaccination, the proportion of immune children 24 months following immunization was only 75%, thus 25% of children were susceptible to mumps. Although the rate of immunogenicity is good, it is not high enough to reach herd immunity of 95%.
- If such finding are confirmed in further larger studies, a booster dose of mumps vaccine in children very soon after vaccination (e.g. 1–2 months) (due to 14% vaccine failure) or 2 years after the first vaccination (due to level of immunity decreasing to 75% at this time) may be suggested.
- This study is in line with the Ministry of Health and Education's strategy to conduct a nationwide survey to confirm level of immunity, and to change the strain of mumps included in the MMR vaccine in the Islamic Republic of Iran.

for mumps immunoglobulin M (IgM) and immunoglobulin G (IgG) by enzyme-linked immunosorbent assay (ELISA) (kits manufactured by Trinity Biotech Capita, Jamestown, NY).

Statistical analysis was performed based on the Statistical Package for Social Sciences (SPSS), version 11.5. By using the Fisher exact test, MacNemar test and chi square test, *P* values less than 0.05 were considered statistically significant. Owing to nearly 100% seronegativity of IgM3 after 12 months, the IgM4 test was not checked at 24 months.

Main study findings

Of the 338 children screened for mumps IgG antibody by ELISA method, 14.5% reported previous vaccination against mumps. A total of 67 (19.8%) were mumps IgG negative, indicating that they were susceptible; about 23% of girls tested were mumps IgG negative compared with 17.5% of boys tested. Age-specific mumps IgG seroprevalence rose rapidly from 66.7% at age group 7–11 years (primary schools) to 79.5% at age group 12–14 years (guidance schools) to 95.4% at age group 15–18 years (high schools). Using χ^2, there was a statistically significant difference between age and seroprevalence ($P < 0.05$).

Forty-four (44) mumps IgG-negative subjects accepted the MMR vaccine to evaluate the immunogenicity of the mumps Hoshino strain included in the MMR vaccine. Forty (40) children continued till the end of study and, of those, four (10%) were excluded due to seroconversion (new infection), therefore 36 children successfully completed the study. Blood was collected by venipuncture 3, 12 and 4 months following vaccination and serum samples were tested by ELISA for the detection of mumps IgM and IgG. The overall seroconversion rate was 86.1%, 77.7% and 75% at 3, 12 and 24 months, respectively. The seroconversion rate for the 6–11 year-old age group was 85% at 3 months. Mumps IgG was detected in 75% at 12 months and 24 months postvaccination. Based on the MacNemar test, there was no significant difference. The seroconversion rate for the 12–14 year-old age group was 87.5% at 3 months. Mumps IgG was detected in 81.25% and 75% at 12 months and 24 months postvaccination, respectively. The difference was not statistically significant. Two subjects developed parotiditis and fever, 7–31 days following vaccination; this was confirmed by serology.

Conclusions and recommendations

The study reported a 86% seroconversion rate following postvaccination of the Hoshino strain of mumps, which is included in the MMR vaccine. This indicates that the vaccine failure rate was about 14%. A steady decline in the proportion of immune children was observed when tested at 3, 12 and 24 months after receiving the vaccine. The proportion of immune children 24 months following immunization was 75%, and 25% of the children tested remained non-immune and susceptible.

Diagnosis

Sudan

Visceral leishmaniasis

Evaluation of the 2-mercaptoethanol enzyme-linked immunosorbent assay (ELISA) for improved diagnosis of visceral leishmaniasis in endemic eastern Sudan

- **Sudan**
  Doka Gedaref State
- **Study period**
  November 2005–
  November 2006
- **Small Grants Scheme**
  (SGS) 2005 No. 146
- **Principal Investigator**
  Durria Mansour Elhussein
  Biomedical Research Laboratory
  Ahfad University for Women
  Omdurman, Sudan
  e-mail: durriaelhussein@hotmail.com

Abstract

An evaluation was carried out of a newly developed 2-mercaptoethanol (2-ME) enzyme-linked immunosorbent assay (ELISA) for detection of visceral leishmaniasis (VL). A total of 322 patients with VL were enrolled. The 2-ME immunoglobulin G (IgG) ELISA and the direct agglutination test (DAT) were applied to sera collected from all parasitologically confirmed (125 persons) and clinically VL suspects (197 persons). Results were compared with those of two groups of apparently healthy individuals from the same endemic area (56 persons) or from Khartoum State (39 persons), a non-endemic area.

Results A total of 114/125 of parasitologically confirmed VL cases scored positive readings in 2-ME IgG ELISA (absorbance: 0.14–1.58) as well as in DAT (titres 1:100 to 1: ≥ 102 400), implying 92.2% sensitivity for both tests. In the 197 clinically VL suspects, discrepant results were obtained in 8 patients (4.1%). Irrespective of the area chosen, specificity of 2-ME IgG ELISA in the apparently healthy individuals was similar to DAT (98.2% versus 100%). The incorporation of IgM conjugate in the newly developed 2-ME ELISA for monitoring of early VL was less successful, as the levels measured for this immunoglobulin class were not different ($P \geq 0.168$) from those obtained in the apparently healthy controls. Despite the noticeable clinical improvement after completion of antileishmanial treatment, 2-ME ELISA absorbance values remained almost the same on days 0, 10, 20 and 30. However, the performance of DAT was slightly better, as 4 out of 27 treated patients showed a fourfold dilution decline 30 days after start of treatment.

Conclusion The 2-ME ELISA demonstrated a high diagnostic efficiency, supporting the recommendation of its use as a complementary test for VL diagnosis in moderately equipped laboratories.

Background

Visceral leishmaniasis (VL) is among the most important health problems in Sudan. More than 24 660 cases and 1193 deaths were reported during 1996–2001 [1]. Early diagnosis of VL is important in order to avoid severe health damage or even death. Routine diagnosis relies either on microscopic demonstration of *Leishmania* amastigotes in organ aspirates (lymph nodes, bone marrow or spleen) or on in vitro parasite culturing. As these techniques are invasive and time consuming, the development of easy, rapid and non-invasive methods would be valuable. Despite high reliability for diagnosis, marginal titres were occasionally recorded for the direct agglutination test (DAT) in non-VL patients [2]. As an alternative to the conventional water-soluble antigen, an intact promastigote antigen treated with 2-mercaptoethanol (2-ME) has been evaluated in enzyme-linked immunosorbent assay (ELISA) for the detection of antileishmanial immunoglobulin G (IgG) antibodies [3]. In this study, the performance of 2-ME ELISA was evaluated and compared with DAT in a known VL-endemic area in eastern Sudan.

Conclusions and implications of the study

- Performance of the newly developed 2-ME ELISA at laboratory level was highly concordant with results obtained by DAT.
- A comparable high diagnostic efficiency (sensitivity 92.2% and specificity 98.2%) was also demonstrated in this study. These results provide further support for the recommendation of 2-ME ELISA as a complementary test for VL diagnosis in moderately equipped laboratories, such as those found in Sudan.
- In addition to the high sensitivity and specificity, 2-ME ELISA has additional advantages compared with DAT. The antigen requires significantly fewer numbers of promastigotes (2.5 x 107/ml) than required by DAT (5.0 x 107/ml). In addition, reading of the test reaction can be performed within 4 h, compared with 18 h in DAT. If antigen-precoated plates are used, execution and reading of the test results can be achieved within 3 h.
- IgM levels were indistinguishable from those of healthy individuals from endemic or non-endemic areas.

Materials and methods

A comparative cross-sectional study was carried out to evaluate the efficiency of 2-ME ELISA and DAT for diagnosis of VL in the Doka area, eastern Sudan. Three hundred and twenty two (322) clinically suspected VL cases were reported to the rural hospital in Doka. Of those, 125 were parasitologically confirmed VL cases, while 197 were negative with high suspicion for VL. All patients and their guardians agreed to participate in the study. Clinical data and patient characteristics were collected using a standard form detailing sex, age, weight, clinical complaints, physical examination, and results of laboratory investigations, including DAT and 2-ME ELISA. Treated VL patients underwent clinical and serological 10-day interval follow-up for 1 month. Other laboratory tests were also performed, including blood film for malaria and sputum for acid-fast bacilli. Treated VL patients were also assessed for intercurrent infections and post-treatment complications. A group of apparently healthy volunteers (*n* = 95) was included in the study to serve as controls.

Main study findings

Of the 322 VL suspects examined, 125 (38.8%) revealed *Leishmania* amastigotes in lymph-node or bone-marrow aspirates. Of the 125 parasitologically confirmed VL patients tested, 114 (91.2%) were positive at 2-ME ELISA; the same sensitivity was demonstrated by DAT. Eleven (11) samples gave negative absorbance values below the cut-off (0.29) at the range of 0.14–0.27. No cross-reaction (0.11–0.28) was observed in the non-endemics (*n* = 39), implying 100% specificity for 2-ME ELISA. One out of 56 endemic healthy individuals scored an absorbance value of 0.36. Specificity of 2-ME ELISA was therefore 98.2% in this population. As for 2-ME ELISA, no cross-reaction was demonstrated for DAT in the endemic or non-endemic populations, showing 100% specificity. A high degree of concordance (96.8%) was found between the two tests in the confirmed VL patient group. Despite this high concordance, discrepancies were noticed in 8 of the VL suspects. Among 197 patients with high suspicion for VL, both tests gave positive readings in 15 (7.6%) patients. In 7 patients (3.6%), while 2-ME ELISA scored positive, results of DAT were negative. Despite the difference, concordance between the two tests in this population was excellent (94.9%). No significant differences in IgM levels were found between the VL suspects and the healthy controls.

On the basis of these results, it seems that serum IgM is of less importance in VL diagnosis employing 2-ME-treated promastigote antigen. Neither 2-ME ELISA nor DAT can be used as a follow-up procedure for VL during treatment or shortly after its completion.

Conclusions and recommendations

Performance of the developed 2-ME ELISA at laboratory level was highly concordant with results obtained by DAT. These results provide further support to the recommendation for applying 2-ME ELISA as a complementary test for VL diagnosis in moderately equipped laboratories, such as those found in the Sudan.

References

[1] Ministry of Health. *Manual for diagnosis and treatment.* Sudan, Ministry of Health, 2003.

[2] Harith AE et al. Improvement of a direct agglutination test for field studies of visceral leishmaniasis. *Journal of Clinical Microbiology*, 1988, 26:1321–1325.

[3] Abass EM, Mansour D, el Motasim M et al. ß-Mercaptoethanol-modified ELISA for diagnosis of visceral leishmaniasis. *Journal of Medical Microbiology*, 2006, 55: 1193–1196.

Visceral leishmaniasis

Evaluation of a non-invasive antigen-based ELISA assay for diagnosis of visceral leishmaniasis

- **Islamic Republic of Iran**
- **Study period**
  2005–2006

- **Small Grants Scheme**
  (SGS) 2005 No. 62

- **Principal Investigator**
  Bahador Sarkari
  Faculty of Medicine
  Yasuj University of Medical Sciences
  Yasuj, Islamic Republic of Iran
  e-mail: sarkarib@yahoo.com

Abstract

A non-invasive antigen-based enzyme-linked immunosorbent assay (ELISA) system was evaluated for diagnosis of visceral leishmaniasis (VL). Urine samples from confirmed VL cases were tested by this system and compared with urine samples from patients with non-VL infectious disease and patients with non-infectious diseases.

Results Antigen was detected in the urine of 21 out of 35 (60%) of VL cases. No cross-reaction was found with samples from healthy individuals, while three samples from non-VL infectious diseases (two samples from a cutaneous leishmaniasis patient and one from a patient with toxoplasmosis) were found to be positive by this system. The antigen-based ELISA results were compared with those obtained from a direct agglutination test (DAT), an antibody-based ELISA and an indirect immunofluorescent antibody test (IFAT). The antigen-based ELISA was comparable in term of specificity (91.2%) but had lower sensitivity (60%).

Conclusion These results suggest that antigen detection in urine by the non-invasive antigen-based ELISA system may offer a useful method for diagnosis of VL.

Background

Visceral leishmaniasis (VL) is a serious public health problem in many tropical and subtropical regions of the world, including the Islamic Republic of Iran. Parasitological diagnosis of VL is still a routine method of diagnosis. However, it is an invasive and risky method and its sensitivity is estimated to be about 50–85% [1]. Moreover, parasitological diagnosis is not a field-applicable method and cannot be used for epidemiological studies. A number of serological techniques have been developed for diagnosis of VL, including enzyme-linked immunosorbent assay (ELISA), dot ELISA and direct agglutination test (DAT). The sensitivity and specificity of such diagnostic methods depend on the type, source and purity of the antigen employed.

An alternative to antibody detection is antigen detection in urine or serum, which is a recent approach in the diagnosis of parasitic infections. Recent work in the field of antigen detection in leishmaniasis resulted in the demonstration of an antigen in the urine of VL patients by a latex agglutination test ("Katex") [2]. The sensitivity and specificity of Katex was found to be 70–80% and 100%, respectively, if the sample was boiled for 5 min before testing. Further work showed that the target antigen for this agglutination test is a low molecular weight (5–20 kDa) carbohydrate antigen [3]. The current study was performed using a non-invasive antigen-based ELISA assay for diagnosis of VL using urine samples.

Materials and methods

A bone marrow sample was taken from a 5-year-old child suspected of VL. The sample was cultured in biphasic blood agar medium and then transferred to RPMI 1640 with 10% fetal calf serum (FCS) for mass cultivation. To determine the species of parasite, isoenzyme and polymerase chain reaction (PCR) (semi-nested PCR) techniques were performed. Cultivated parasite was used for rabbit immunization for production of anti-*Leishmania* antibody. A total of 61 serum

Conclusions and implications of the study

- Serological methods are mostly based on the detection of antibodies in serum. A number of serological tests, including IFAT, ELISA and DAT, have provided a relatively good efficacy in diagnosis of VL.
- This study evaluated the usefulness of an antigen-based capture ELISA for diagnosis of VL. Results showed that this system has a relatively high specificity for diagnosis of VL.
- A good PPV was found for this assay. When the results of capture ELISA were compared with routine antibody-detection assays (indirect ELISA, DAT and IFAT), a high specificity was found for capture ELISA, while the highest sensitivity was found for indirect ELISA.
- The capture ELISA uses urine specimens, rather than serum, which reduces the risk of infection to the person carrying out the test.

and 35 urine samples were collected from VL patients from Fars and Kohgiluyeh and Boyerahmad provinces. In addition, 34 urine samples were taken from healthy controls and from patients with different microbial infections, but not VL. DAT was performed on serum of VL patients and also control samples, to compare the efficacy of this well-known test with the antigen-based ELISA. The indirect immunofluorescent antibody test (IFAT) was performed using formalin-washed promastigote of *Leishmania infantum*.

Main study findings

Among the studied cases, 80.3% of patients had a positive IFAT while 38.5% had a positive parasitological test using bone marrow aspiration. Bone marrow aspiration was not performed in all cases. DAT showed a sensitivity of 70.5% (good) and a specificity of 100%. Positive predictive value (PPV) and negative predictive value (NPV) were 100% and 74.6%, respectively, for this assay. A significant agreement (61.5%) was found between DAT and direct parasitological tests.

When the serum samples were tested by an ELISA system, using crude *L. infantum* antigen, a sensitivity of 83.6 (95% confidence interval, CI = 71.4–91.4) and specificity of 83.6 (95% CI = 78.6–96.5) was found for this assay. PPV and NPV of 91.5% (95% CI = 79.6–96.7) and 82.7 (95% CI = 70.1–91) was calculated for this assay. An agreement rate of 48% was found between ELISA and bone marrow examination. The urine samples were tested for detection of leishmanial urinary antigen. The samples were 35 from VL cases and 34 samples with cutaneous leishmaniasis, toxoplasmosis, brucellosis, malaria and hydatidosis) and also healthy subjects. Antigen from non-VL patients (from patients was detected in urine of 21 from 35 cases of VL patients. While none of the healthy individuals gave a positive reaction in the assay, three sample from non-VL patients, one from a toxoplasmosis patient and two samples from cutaneous leishmaniasis patients, had a false-positive reaction with this system. Having these, a sensitivity of 60% (95% CI = 42.4–75.6) was calculated for the antigen detection assay. PPV and NPV of 87.5 (95% CI = 66.5–96.5) and 68.9 (95% CI = 53.2–81.4) was calculated for the assay. A significant agreement rate (41.1%) was found between this assay and direct parasitological examination using bone marrow aspiration. The system also had a reasonable agreement (51.4%) with DAT and indirect ELISA (54.3%), using serum sample.

Conclusions and recommendations

The newly introduced antigen-detection ELISA assay might be a good alternative to routine antibody-detection assays, especially where a high level of antigen is expected, i.e. in *Leishmania*/HIV coinfected patients.

References

[1] Berman J. Recent developments in leishmaniasis: epidemiology, diagnosis, and treatment. *Current Infectious Disease Reports*, 2005, 7:33–38.

[2] Attar ZJ et al. Latex agglutination test for the detection of urinary antigens in visceral leishmaniasis. *Acta Tropica*, 2001, 78:11–16.

[3] Sarkari B, Chance M, Hommel M. Antigenuria in visceral leishmaniasis: detection and partial characterisation of a carbohydrate antigen. *Acta Tropica*, 2002, 82:339–348.

Visceral leishmaniasis

Seroconversion and induction of the leishmanin skin test in healthy Sudanese living in the kala-azar endemic area in eastern Sudan

- **Sudan**
  Gadarif State
- **Study period**
  November 2005–November 2006

- **Small Grants Scheme**
  (SGS) 2005 No. 99

- **Principal Investigator**
  El Waleed ElAmin
  Institute of Endemic Diseases
  University of Khartoum
  Khartoum, Sudan
  e-mail: wmelamin@hotmail.com

Abstract

A longitudinal study was carried out in a leishmaniasis-endemic region in eastern Sudan. The objectives of the study were to monitor the seroconversion, leishmanin skin test (LST) induction and asymptomatic infections in villagers living in endemic area with visceral leishmaniasis (VL) by repeated surveys every 4 months. The transmission of infection was monitored by measuring the vector density and the rate of infection of the vector. A sample of 700 healthy volunteers was selected for the study. All participants were subjected to the direct agglutination test (DAT) and also LST screening. In addition, kDNA/polymerase chain reaction (PCR) was used for detection of asymptomatic parasitaemia in the blood.

Results The results obtained showed insignificant DAT and LST conversion during the study period. No *Leishmania* DNA was detected using kDNA/PCR amplification of collected blood samples. Furthermore, no infected sand flies were found in the area although the density was not low. In addition, none of the volunteers developed symptoms of VL during the study period.

Conclusion The overall data indicated the absence or very low transmission of *Leishmania* infection in the village during the study period.

Background

Leishmaniasis is a group of diseases, caused by protozoan haemoflagellated parasites of the genus *Leishmania* and presenting in different clinical forms. Visceral leishmaniasis (VL), which is the most serious form of the disease, is characterized by the development of fever, splenomegaly, hepatomegaly, weight loss and pancytopenia. The infection is fatal if not treated, and may be complicated by epistaxis, concurrent infections or post-kala-azar dermal leishmaniasis (PKDL).

Different forms of leishmaniasis are endemic in Sudan and pose serious health problems [1]. Sudan is one of five countries where 90% of new VL cases occur [2]. The sand-fly vector for VL in Sudan was previously reported as *Phlebotomus orientalis* [3]. Frequent epidemics of the visceral form of leishmaniasis in Sudan claimed hundreds of thousands of lives [4]. Three regions are known to be endemic for VL: the eastern region including the vital agricultural area in Gadaref State, the central region of the Blue Nile State and the southern region of the Upper Nile State [1]. The role of asymptomatic patients in parasite transmission is not known. Early detection of asymptomatic cases will result in the early treatment of such cases and in better control of the disease.

Conclusions and implications of the study

- The absence of infection in sand flies may be due to low, or no, transmission of leishmaniasis in the area during these months, or may be due to the fact that most flies emerging at the beginning of the vector season were nulliparous.
- The high rate of negative results of the LST indicated a low transmission pattern of *Leishmania* infection in the village during the study period. The low LST conversion is supported by entomology results conducted during the same period in the village, which showed low catching rate of sand fly.
- In this study, about 5% of participants showed positive DAT results although none had a history of treated kala-azar or even cutaneous leishmaniasis infection. Most probably, these results are due to exposure of the participants to *Leishmania* infection (asymptomatic infection). The mechanisms implicated in susceptibility in humans are not fully understood.
- The low densities of *Phlebotomus papatasi* and *P. orientalis* during the present study may be a result of meteorological or other ecological changes. This finding is important, as it could result in a corresponding increase in the risk of acquiring kala-azar within the villages of the endemic region.

The main objective of this study was to monitor the direct agglutination test (DAT), leishmanin skin test (LST) conversion and asymptomatic infections of villagers living in a kala-azar endemic area in Gadarif state, eastern Sudan as indicators for the development of clinical VL.

Materials and methods

A longitudinal study was conducted in a leishmaniasis-endemic area. A sample of 700 consenting healthy volunteers was randomly selected and recruited. The inclusion criteria were: living in the village; healthy; with no history of kala-azar or PKDL; and no history of kala-azar treatment. Children were preferred, as they present a vulnerable group and usually do not travel out of the village. For each volunteer, a questionnaire was completed in the first survey to collect baseline data such as age, gender, tribe, name of head of the tribe (sheikh) and detailed description of residence. All participants were subjected to clinical examination at the beginning of the study. Repeated DAT, LST and kDNA/polymerase chain reaction (PCR) surveys were conducted every 4 months.

Main study findings

The 700 consenting volunteers in this study were included in the first field survey; 620 of these volunteers were then followed in the second and 485 in the third field survey. Among the studied group, 618 were young, with ages ranging from 6 to 15 years. The male/female ratio was 1:1.5. Results of LSTs showed 37 seroconversions in the first survey, 24 in the second and 23 in the third, with no significant conversion but with significant correlation between the survey results. The same results were obtained for DATs.

A total number of 3002 sand flies were caught in the three field visits during the study period. Three *Phlebotomus* species and five *Sergentomyia* species were dissected. No flies were infected. The PCR results of the screened samples collected in the three field visits showed no circulating *Leishmania* DNA.

Conclusions and recommendations

No significant DAT or LST conversion was detected among the studied group. In addition, few *P. orientalis* vectors were detected and none was infected. Furthermore, no clinical VL developed among the studied group. The overall data indicated absence or very low transmission of *Leishmania* infection in the village during the period of the study.

References

[1] El Hassan AM, Zijlstra E. Leishmaniasis in the Sudan. *Transactions of the Royal Society of Tropical Medicine and Hygiene*, 2001, 95(Suppl. 1), S1–S75.

[2] Fact Sheet No. 116, revised May 2000. Geneva, World Health Organization, 2000.

[3] Elnaiem DA et al. Infection rates of *Leishmania donovani* in *Phlebotomas orientalis* from a focus of visceral leishmaniasis in eastern Sudan. *Annals of Tropical Medicine and Parasitology*, 1998, 92:877–887.

[4] Ashford RW et al. Epidemic visceral leishmaniasis in southern Sudan: identity and systematic position of the parasites from patients and vectors. *Transactions of the Royal Society of Tropical Medicine and Hygiene*, 1992, 86:379–380.

Visceral leishmaniasis

Development of a geographic information system to inform surveillance and control activities for visceral leishmaniasis and other vector-borne and/or zoonotic diseases in north-west Islamic Republic of Iran

- **Islamic Republic of Iran**
  East Azerbaijan Province
- **Study period**
  2006–2007
- **Small Grants Scheme**
  (SGS) 2006 No. 89

- **Principal Investigator**
  Abdolsalam Mazloumi Gavgani
  Department of Medical Parasitology
  Drug Applied Research Center
  Tabriz University of Medical Sciences
  Tabriz, Iran
  e-mail: mazloumi@tbzmed.ac.ir

Abstract

Visceral leishmaniasis (VL) is an increasing and spreading public health problem in the Islamic Republic of Iran, especially in the north-west of the country. A study was developed for mapping the distribution and occurrence of VL in north-west Islamic Republic of Iran in relation to different environmental factors. Geographical information systems (GIS) were used to extract and map for environmental variables, topographic variation, socioeconomic impact, lifestyle, village environment effect and individual factors.

Results The study found that average rainfall, altitude, distance from river, age, nomadic lifestyle and dog abundance were the best predictors of VL incidence. People most at risk included dog owners and nomads. The annual average occurrence of VL disease per whole area was about 1.4/1000 population. All ages and both genders are at equal risk of infection, although the risk that infection leads to disease decreases rapidly with age. Almost all VL patients were less than 10 years old.

Conclusion Findings of this study are relevant to the planning of effective control strategies for VL in north-west Islamic Republic of Iran.

Background

Visceral leishmaniasis (VL) is currently sporadic in 31 provinces of the Islamic Republic of Iran and endemic at least in six provinces. There is a need to develop a better understanding of the spatiotemporal patterns in the demographics and epidemiology of humans and animals, and the spatial synchrony between these populations. In this project, available medical village-level data were integrated into a geographical information system (GIS), incorporating demographic, socioeconomic, environmental and health-care access data. Village locations were determined using global positioning systems. The above databases and spatial platforms provided a unique opportunity for determining the spatiotemporal distribution of human VL and the

Conclusions and implications of the study

- In this study, current maps of VL in Kalaybar and Ahar districts, important endemic regions in north-west Islamic Republic of Iran, were analysed in relation to Ministry of Health-reported cases of VL and data from large-scale prospective epidemiological and diagnostic (MST and DAT) surveys in Kalaybar and Ahar districts. More than 10 000 individuals were sampled and some of the results obtained from the epidemiological survey were used in interpretations of the maps.
- Results showed that distance from the river, topography, rainfall, temperature and low altitude are the main geographical variables associated with the distribution and incidence of VL in Kalaybar and Ahar districts. It is probable that these variables influence the populations of the vector and the reservoir hosts of L. infantum by affecting other microclimatic factors in the area.
- The strong relationship detected between the transmission rate in humans and dogs in different villages provides further evidence for the role of infected dogs in the transmission of VL to humans.
- In general, a large number of phlebotomine sand flies were observed in the regions associated with many cases of canine and human leishmaniasis; this should be given priority in leishmaniasis-control measures.
- The study results also indicated significant association between nomadic living condition and incidence of disease. The highlighted factors in nomadic living conditions were movement in endemic areas and ownership of several dogs.
- In villages with health centres, there seemed to be a direct relationship between health education and policy by health staff, and changes in the behaviour of the population and in the environment, which could lead to a reduction in transmission rate of the infection.

relationship with animal demography and epidemiology. Spatial clustering and time–space clustering of disease cases and spatial synchrony in human demography and epidemiology were explored. An important longer-term aim of this work was to incorporate a spatiotemporal dimension into analytical frameworks that seek to describe transmission dynamics of VL, and to explore the cost effectiveness of different control interventions.

Materials and methods

The study was developed for mapping the distribution and occurrence of VL in north-west Islamic Republic of Iran in relation to different environmental factors. GIS was used to extract and map for environmental variables for all villages in Kalaybar and Ahar districts, including climate variation (average temperature and rainfall of 10 years), topographic variation (altitude and distance from river), socioeconomic impact (village facilities, presence of health centre), lifestyle and village environmental effect (nomadic condition, dog abundance ownership), and individual factors (age, gender, symptoms, dog ownership). VL occurrence in each village was calculated from Ministry of Health records. Using logistic and linear multivariate regression analyses, models were developed to determine which environmental factors explain variability in the presence and incidence of VL.

Main study findings

The estimated cumulative Montenegro skin test (MST) prevalence and seroprevalence, determined by the direct agglutination test (DAT) of *Leishmania infantum* infection in the total population were 19.7% and 4.7%, respectively. Since 1980, the mean force of infection was estimated to be 2.8% per year, and from 1995 to 1996 it was between 2.2% and 2.6% per year. A marked variation in VL incidence per thousand people was observed between different villages in relation to time. Patients were mostly children; 73% of the cases were under 2 years and almost 96% were under 10 years. The general distribution of VL of endemic and non-endemic villages in relation to altitude showed clear clustering of high occurrence at villages in low altitude and low rainfall and moderate temperature zones. A significant effect of the river on presence of VL was obvious. This may be a reflection of the effect of climate on vectors and reservoirs. The probability of occurrence of VL in a village appeared to be significantly negatively correlated with the rainfall average above 500 mm.

VL cases in males were more common than in females, which may be associated with dressing patterns in each gender affecting exposure to sand flies. It may also be due to more exposure of males to sand flies due to occupation. Reported VL cases occurred in districts mostly far from the health centres. Health-post presence may have an impact on efficiency of control programmes and on environmental and individual behavioural changes. Distribution of the disease cases was not related to population density. The strong relationship detected between the transmission rate in humans and dogs in different villages provides further evidence for the role of infected dogs in the transmission of VL to humans. There were big reductions in VL cases following the use of insecticide-impregnated dog collars during 1997–2006.

Conclusions and recommendations

This study provides estimates for various parameters of *L. infantum* infection in humans, including risk factors for infection at the individual or village level, effects of climate and geographical variations, effect of reservoir host and vectors and socioeconomic factors.

Visceral leishmaniasis

Development and evaluation of an rK39 plus rK26 ELISA test for serodiagnosis of visceral leishmaniasis caused by *Leishmania infantum* in an endemic area of the Islamic Republic of Iran

- **Islamic Republic of Iran**
- **Study period**
  2005–2006

- **Small Grants Scheme**
  (SGS) 2005 No.95

- **Principal Investigator**
  Safar Farajnia
  Drug Applied Research Center
  Tabriz University of Medical Science
  Tabriz, Islamic Republic of Iran
  e-mail: farajnia@yahoo.com

Abstract

Human visceral leishmaniasis (VL), caused by *Leishmania infantum*, is a severe health problem in the Middle East and in many Mediterranean basin countries. Reliable diagnosis is essential to prevent mortality and morbidity due to VL. The purpose of this study was to prepare recombinant K39 and K26 antigens from *L. infantum* and to evaluate their performance in an enzyme-linked immunosorbent assay (ELISA) test for serodiagnosis of VL in endemic regions of the Islamic Republic of Iran. Sera from 617 subjects, including 187 patients with confirmed VL, 30 patients with other common infectious diseases, 200 healthy controls and 200 recovered cases, were tested.

Results The rK39-rK26 ELISA was positive in 184 of 187 patients with confirmed *L. infantum* infection (sensitivity = 98.4%) and negative in 230 of 230 subjects who either had other disease or were healthy (specificity = 100%). In comparison, the direct agglutination test (DAT) was positive in 181 of 187 VL patients (sensitivity = 90.9%) and negative in 211 of 230 subjects who either had other diseases or were healthy (specificity = 89%).

Conclusion The results of this study indicated that the rK39-rK26 ELISA is a sensitive and specific test for the serodiagnosis of VL and could be used for reliable diagnosis of VL caused by *L. infantum*.

Background

Visceral leishmaniasis (VL), or kala-azar, is a potentially fatal disease caused by a protozoan parasite of the *Leishmania donovani* complex. Zoonotic VL is endemic in north-western and central parts of the Islamic Republic of Iran and caused by *Leishmania infantum*. Classically, the diagnosis of VL is made by demonstration of *Leishmania* amastigotes in aspirates from lymph nodes, bone marrow or spleen. However, these techniques are invasive, require skilled personnel and well-equipped hospitals and are limited by their low sensitivity. The direct agglutination test (DAT) is popular in most countries but variation between batches of antigen and cross-reaction with other infectious agents are limiting factors. Furthermore, the test may remain positive for several years after a patient is cured and thus does not distinguish between past and present infection. Different recombinant antigens have been tested for serodiagnosis of VL and rK39 and rK26 antigens have shown promising results in different studies.

The objective of this study was to clone and characterize *L. infantum* K39 and K26 antigens and to evaluate their performance in serodiagnosis of VL caused by *L. infantum* in endemic region of the Islamic Republic of Iran.

Materials and methods

Sera were screened from four different groups. Group A comprised 187 patients with active VL, randomly selected from diagnosed patients referred to the children's hospital of Tabriz, children's hospital of Ardabil or rural health-care

Conclusions and implications of the study

- The currently used method of laboratory diagnosis is based on finding the parasite in bone-marrow biopsy or spleen aspiration. This invasive method is not applicable in most rural settings. Furthermore, it has low sensitivity.
- Serological methods have proven to be useful non-invasive methods for the rapid diagnosis of VL. In addition, these methods could have epidemiological applications for determining carrier rates among asymptomatic subjects and could also be used to map out the geographical distribution of the infection.
- These results confirm that the combination of rK26 and rK39 antigens improves the sensitivity of the test without any decline in specificity. Another important facet of K39 antigen is that the titre of antibody against this antigen correlates with the disease activity.

centres. Group B comprised 200 patients who had been treated for VL in the past 3 years and had recovered, randomly selected from patient files in the hospital of Tabriz, Ardabil or health-care centres. Group C comprised 200 healthy controls, with no history of leishmaniasis, randomly selected from cities in endemic regions such as the central part of Tehran and Tabriz city. Group D comprised 10 tuberculosis, 10 brucellosis and 10 toxoplasmosis patients, randomly selected from the same health facilities. All patients were from East Azerbaijan and Ardabil provinces in north-west Islamic Republic of Iran, where VL is endemic.

The following procedures were performed on the collected specimens: preparation of DNA, polymerase chain reaction (PCR) amplification of *L. infantum* k39 and k26 genes; cloning of PCR products and DNA sequencing; and expression and purification of recombinant Li-k39. The ELISA test was carried out according to the standard method with slight modification. The direct agglutination test (DAT) was also performed.

Main study findings

The rk39 ELISA was positive for 179 out of 187 patients, giving a sensitivity of 95.7%. The rk26 ELISA was positive for 178 of 187 patients, giving a sensitivity of 95.2%. The rk39 plus rk26 ELISA was positive for 184 of 187 patients, giving a sensitivity of 98.4%. The whole-cell ELISA and DAT were positive for 181 of 187 patients and 171 of 187 patients of VL sera, giving a sensitivity of 96.8% and 1.4%, respectively. The rK39 ELISA, rK26 ELISA and rK39-rK26 ELISA gave negative results for 200 of 200 healthy controls and for all 30 samples from other infectious diseases, giving a specificity of 100%. In contrast, the DAT and whole-cell ELISA produced false-positive results for 24 of 230 and 27 of 230 non-VL subjects, giving a specificity of 89.6% and 88.3%, respectively.

Conclusions and recommendations

The study reported the validity of the rK39-rK26 ELISA as a sensitive and specific test for the diagnosis of VL caused by *L. infantum*. The test reported a higher sensitivity and specificity compared to DAT (98.4% and 100%, versus 90.9% and 89%, respectively). The results of this study showed that both K39 and K26 are highly reactive and diagnostically valuable antigens. The sensitivity obtained by rK39 + rK26 antigens was higher than that of single antigen, which indicates the complementary effects of these two antigens; this could be used to enhance the sensitivity of the serodiagnostic test.

List of publications

Articles originating from the Small Grants Scheme supported projects 1992–2008

1 Kamhawi A, et al. Environmental manipulation in the control of a zoonotic cutaneous leishmaniasis focus. *Archive de L'Institut* Pasteur de Tunis, 1993, 70(3–4):383–90.

2 Moukrim A, Zekhnini A, Rondelaud D. Observations écologiques sur les hôtes ntermédiaires de *Schistosoma haematobium* Bilharz dans la province d'Agadir (Maroc). *Bulletin de la Société Française de Parasitologie*, 1993, 11(2):223–30.

3 Zekhnini A, Mansir A, Moukrim A. Nouvelles données sur les hôtes intermédiaires de *Schistosoma haematobium* dans la province d'Agadir (Maroc). La pénétration du miracidum et son devenir chez trois pulmones. *Bulletin de la Société Française de Parasitologie*, 1993, 11(1):85–94.

4 Arbaji AK, Gradoni L, Gramiccia M. Leishmanin skin test survey in a focus of high endemicity of *Leishmania major* in Jordan. *Acta tropica*, 1993, 54(1):77–9.

5 Al-Haddad AM. Research Abstract. New foci of schistosomiasis transmission in Yemen. *Eastern Mediterranean health journal*, 1995, 1(2):294–96.

6 Janini R, et al. Incrimination of *Phlebotomus papatasi* as vector of *Leishmania major* in the southern Jordan Valley. *Medical and veterinary entomology*, 1995, 9(4):420–22.

7 Hilali AH, et al. Infection and transmission pattern of *Schistosoma mansoni* in the Managil irrigation scheme, Sudan. *Annals of tropical medicine and parasitology*, 1995, 89(3):279–86.

8 Baraka OZ, et al. Community based distribution of ivermectin in eastern Sudan: acceptability and early post-treatment reactions. *Transactions of the Royal Society of Tropical Medicine and Hygiene*, 1995, 89(3):316–18.

9 Baraka OZ, et al. Ivermectin treatment in severe asymmetric reactive onchodermatitis (sowda) in Sudan. *Transactions of the Royal Society of Tropical Medicine and Hygiene*, 1995, 89(3):312–15.

10 Attallah AM, El-Masry SA. Detection of circulating antigens in individuals infected with schistosomiasis using monoclonal antibodies and fast dot-ELISA. *Eastern Mediterranean health journal*, 1996, 2(2):340.

11 Farag H. Evaluation of an integrated approach to schistosomiasis control in a resettlement area west of Alexandria. *Eastern Mediterranean health journal*, 1996, 2(3):558–59.

12 Hammad TA, et al. Comparative evaluation of the use of artificial neural networks for modeling the epidemiology of *schistosoma mansoni*. T*ransactions of the Royal Society of Tropical Medicine and Hygiene*, 1996, 90(4):372–6.

13 Moukrim A, Zekhnini A, Rondelaud D. *Schistosoma haematobium*: influence of the number of miracidia on several characteristics of infection in newborn *Planorbarius metidjensis. Parasitology research*, 1996, 82(3):267–9.

14 Attallah AM, et al. Fast-dot ELISA using urine, a rapid and dependable field assay for diagnosis of schistosomiasis. *Journal of the Egyptian Society of Parasitology*, 1997, 27(1):279–89.

15 Zekhnini A, et al. *Schistosoma haematobium*: comparative studies on prevalence and cercarial shedding according to the shell diameter of *Planorbarius metidjensis* at miracidial exposure. *Parasitology research*, 1997, 83(3):303–5.

16 Al-Shamahy H. Seroprevalence of kala-azar among humans and dogs in Yemen. Annals of *Saudi medicine*, 1998, 18(1):66–8.

17 Attallah AM, et al. Immunochemical purification and characterization of a 74.0-kDa *Schistosoma mansoni* antigen. *Journal of parasitology*, 1998, 84(2):301–6.

18 Mengad R, et al. Production of direct agglutination test (DAT) antigen and seroprevalence of visceral leishmaniasis in northern Morocco. *Giornale Italiano di medicina tropicale*, 1998, 3(3–4):83–7.

19. Elnaiem DA, et al. Impact of pyrethroid-impregnated curtains on *Phlebotomus papatasi* sandflies indoors at Khartoum, Sudan. *Medical and veterinary entomology*, 1999, 13(2):191–7

20 Attallah AM, et al. Immunochemical characterization and diagnostic potential of a 63-kilodalton *Schistosoma* antigen. *The American journal of tropical medicine and hygiene*, 1999, 60(3):493–7.

21 Attallah AM, et al. Rapid detection of a *Schistosoma mansoni* circulating antigen excreted in urine of infected individuals by using a monoclonal antibody. *Journal of clinical microbiology*, 1999, 37(2):354–7.

22 Ramzy RMR, et al. Field evaluation of a rapid-format kit for the diagnosis of bancroftian filariasis in Egypt. *Eastern Mediterranean health journal*, 1999, 5(5):880–7.

23 Mengad R, et al. Production of direct agglutination test (DAT) antigen and seroprevalence of visceral leishmaniasis in the northern of Morocco. *Eastern Mediterranean health journal*, 1999, 5(5):1091.

24 Yacoubi B, et al. *Schistosoma haematobium*: comparative studies on the characteristics of infection in three populations of *Planorbarius metidjensis* from the Agadir province in South Morocco. *Parasitology research*, 1999, 85(3):239–42.

25 Nagi MA, et al. Epidemiological, clinical and haematological profile of schistosomiasis in Yemen. *Eastern Mediterranean health journal*, 1999, 5(1):177–81.

26 Ghrab J, Bouattour A. Etude experimentale de l'efficacité larvivore de *Gambusia affinis holbrooki* (Girard, 1859) (Poisson-Poecilidae). *Archive de L'Institut Pasteur de Tunis*, 1999, 76(1–4):33–38.

27 Ibrahim ME, et al. Kala-azar in a high transmission focus: an ethnic and geographic dimension. *The American journal of tropical medicine and hygiene*, 1999, 61(6):941–4.

28 Sassi A, et al. Leishmanin skin test lymphoproliferative responses and cytokine production after symptomatic or asymptomatic *Leishmania major* infection in Tunisia. *Clinical and experimental immunology*, 1999, 116(1):127–32.

29 Abou-Basha LM, et al. Hepatic fibrosis due to fascioliasis and/or schistosomiasis in Abis 1 village, Egypt. *Eastern Mediterranean health journal,* 2000, 6(5–6):870–8.

30 Kheir MM, et al. Effects of single-dose praziquantel on morbidity and mortality resulting from intestinal schistosomiasis. *Eastern Mediterranean health journal*,2000, 6(5–6):926–31.

31 Yousif MA, Adeel AA. Antimalarials prescribing patterns in Gezira State: percepts and practices. *Eastern Mediterranean health journal*, 2000, 6(5–6):939–47.

32 Raja'a YA, et al. Schistosomes infection rate in relation to environmental factors in school children *Saudi medical journal,* 2000, 21(7):635–8.

33 Allam AF. Evaluation of different means of control of snail intermediate host of *Schistosoma mansoni*. *Journal of the Egyptian Society of Parasitology*, 2000, 30(2):441–50.

34 Bassiouny HK. Bioenvironmental and meteorological factors related to the persistence of malaria in Fayoum Governorate: a retrospective study. *Eastern Mediterranean health journal,* 2001, 7(6):895–906.

35 Raja'a YA, et al. Some aspects in the control of schistosomiasis and soil-transmitted helminthiasis in Yemeni children. *Saudi medical journal*, 2001, 22(5):428–32.

36 Kamel MI, et al. Impact of type and stage of schistosomiasis on quality of life and productivity of infected workers. *Journal of the Egyptian Society of Parasitology,* 2001, 31(1):153–67.

37 Ghalib HW, et al. Therapeutic efficacy of chloroquine against uncomplicated, *Plasmodium falciparum* malaria in south-western Saudi Arabia. *Annals of tropical medicine and parasitology*, 2001, 95(8):773–9.

38 Jawabreh AO. Risk assessment of cutaneous leishmaniasis in Jericho city during the period 1994–1999. Islah Charitable Social Committee, Jericho, Palestine Ministry of Health, 2001.

39 Yaghoobi-Ershadi MR, et al. Epidemiological study in a new focus of cutaneous leishmaniosis due to *Leishmania major* in Ardestan town, central Iran. *Acta tropica,* 2001, 79(2):115–21.

40 Abou-Basha LM, et al. Performance of IgG avidity in an area endemic for schistosomiasis in Egypt. *Eastern Mediterranean health journal,* 2002, 8(1):172–80.

41 Musa AM, et al. The natural history of Sudanese post-kala-azar dermal leishmaniasis: clinical, immunological and prognostic features. *Annals of tropical medicine and parasitology*, 2002, 96(8):765–72.

42 Gavgani AS, et al. Effect of insecticide-impregnated dog collars on incidence of zoonotic visceral leishmaniasis in Iranian children: a matched-cluster randomised trial. *Lancet*, 2002, 360(9330):374–9.

43 Gavgani AS, et al. Domestic dog ownership in Iran is a risk factor for human infection with *Leishmania infantum*. *The American journal of tropical medicine and hygiene*, 2002, 67(5):511–15.

44 Yaghoobi-Ershadi MR, et al. A new focus of cutaneous leishmaniasis caused by *Leishmania tropica*. *Saudi medical journal*, 2002, 23(3):291–4.

45 Zaki A, et al. Morbidity of schistosomiasis mansoni in rural Alexandria, Egypt. *Journal of the Egyptian Society of Parasitology*, 2003, 33(3):695–710.

46 Elnaiem DE, et al. Risk mapping of visceral leishmaniasis: the role of local variation in rainfall and altitude on the presence and incidence of kala-azar in eastern Sudan. *The American journal of tropical medicine and hygiene,* 2003, 68(1):107.

47 Parvez SD, Al-Wahaibi SS. Comparison of three larviciding options for malaria vector control. *Eastern Mediterranean health journal,* 2003, 9(4):627–36.

48 Saeed IE, Ahmed ES.. Determinants of acquiring malaria among displaced people in Khartoum state, Sudan. *Eastern Mediterranean health journal,* 2003, 9(4):581–92.

49 Yaghoobi-Ershadi MR, et al. Epidemiological study in a new focus of cutaneous leishmaniasis in the Islamic Republic of Iran. *Eastern Mediterranean health journal,* 2003, 9(4):816–26.

50 Elnaiem D-EA, et al. Factors affecting variations in exposure to infections by *Leishmania donovani* in eastern Sudan. *EasternMediterranean health journal,* 2003, 9(4):827–36.

51 El-Safi SH, et al. Field evaluation of latex agglutination test for detecting urinary antigens in visceral leishmaniasis in Sudan. *Eastern Mediterranean health journal,* 2003, 9(4):844–55.

52 Kamel MI, et al. Gender differences in health care utilization and outcome of respiratory tuberculosis in Alexandria. *Eastern Mediterranean health journal,* 2003, 9(4):741–56.

53 Bashour H, Mamaree F. Gender differences and tuberculosis in the Syrian Arab Republic: patients' attitudes, compliance and outcomes. *Eastern Mediterranean health journal,* 2003, 9(4):757–68.

54 Faraj C, et al. Estimation of malaria transmisson in high-risk provinces of Morocco. *Eastern Mediterranean health journal,* 2003, 9(4):542–7.

55 Oshaghi MA, Sedaghat MM, Vatandoost H.. Molecular characterization of the *Anopheles maculipennis* complex in the Islamic Republic of Iran. *Eastern Mediterranean health journal,* 2003, 9(4):659–66.

56 Abdo-Rabbo A. Prescribing rationality and availability of antimalarial drugs in Hajjah, Yemen. *Eastern Mediterranean health journal,* 2003, 9(4):607–17.

57 Malik EM, et al. Stratification of Khartoum urban area by the risk of malaria transmission. *Eastern Mediterranean health journal,* 2003, 9(4):559–69.

58 Khan J, et al.. Tuberculosis diagnosis and treatment practices of private physicians in Karachi, Pakistan. *Eastern Mediterranean health journal,* 2003, 9(4):769–75.

59 Al-Nahhas S, et al.. Visceral leishmaniasis in the Syrian Arab Republic: early detection using rK39. *Eastern Mediterranean health journal,* 2003, 9(4):856–62.

60 Hassan AN, et al. GIS-based prediction of malaria risk in Egypt. Eastern Mediterranean Health Journal, 2003, 9(4):548–58.

61 Mohan A, Nassir H, Niazi A.. Does routine home visiting improve the return rate and outcome of DOTS patients who delay treatment? *Eastern Mediterranean health journal,* 2003, 9(4):702–8.

62 Abdo-Rabbo A. Household survey of treatment of malaria in Hajjah, Yemen. *Eastern Mediterranean health journal,* 2003, 9(4):600–6.

63 Morsy AM, et al. Predictors of treatment failure among tuberculosis patients under DOTS strategy in Egypt. *Eastern Mediterranean health journal,* 2003, 9(4):689–701.

64 Mohamed. AA. Study of larvivorous fish for malaria vector control in Somalia, 2002. *Eastern Mediterranean health journal,* 2003, 9(4):618–26.

65 Niazi AD, Al-Delaimi AM.. Impact of community participation on treatment outcomes and compliance of DOTS patients in Iraq. *Eastern Mediterranean health journal,* 2003, 9(4):709–17.

66 Al-Jawabreh A, et al. Epidemiology of cutaneous leishmaniasis in the endemic area of Jericho, Palestine. *Eastern Mediterranean health journal,* 2003, 9(4):805–815.

67 Awad OM, Shimaila A. Operational use of neem oil as an alternative anopheline larvicide: Part A: laboratory and field efficacy. *Eastern Mediterranean health journal,* 2003, 9(4):637–45.

68 Awad OM. Operational use of neem oil as an alternative anopheline larvicide. Part B: environmental impact and toxicological potential *Eastern Mediterranean health journal,* 2003, 9(4):646–58.

69 Saeed IE, Ahmed ES.. Determinants of malaria mortality among displaced people in Khartoum state, Sudan. *Eastern Mediterranean health journal,* 2003, 9(4):593–9.

70 Elghazali G, et al. *Plasmodium falciparum* infection during pregnancy in an unstable seasonal transmission area in eastern Sudan. *Eastern Mediterranean health journal,* 2003, 9(4):570–80.

71 Farid HA, et al. Filariasis elimination in Egypt: impact of low microfilaraemics as sources of infection for mosquitoes. *Eastern Mediterranean health journal*, 2003, 9(4):863–72.

72 Shah SK, et al. Do private doctors follow national guidelines for managing pulmonary tuberculosis in Pakistan? *Eastern Mediterranean health journal*, 2003, 9(4):776–88.

73 Suleiman BA, et al. Do doctors in north-western Somalia follow the national guidelines for tuberculosis management? *Eastern Mediterranean health journal*, 2003, 9(4):789–95.

74 Shah SA et al. Prevalence of pulmonary tuberculosis in Karachi juvenile jail, Pakistan. *Eastern Mediterranean health journal*, 2003, 9(4):667–74.

75 Al-Kubaisy W, Al-Dulaymi A, Selman. HD. Active tuberculosis among Iraqi schoolchildren with positive skin tests and their household contacts. *Eastern Mediterranean health journal*, 2003, 9(4):675–88.

76 Shirzadi MR, et al. Adherence of the private sector to national tuberculosis guidelines in the Islamic Republic of Iran, 2001–02. *Eastern Mediterranean health journal*, 2003, 9(4):796–804.

77 Abdo MG, et al. Antimony-resistant *Leishmania donovani* in eastern Sudan: incidence and *in vitro* correlation. *Eastern Mediterranean health journal*, 2003, 9(4):837–43.

78 Hashim DS, Al-Kubaisy W, Al Dulayme. A. Knowledge, attitudes and practices survey among health care workers and tuberculosis patients in Iraq. *Eastern Mediterranean health journal*, 2003, 9(4):718–31.

79 Agboatwalla M et al. Gender perspectives on knowledge and practices regarding tuberculosis in urban and rural areas in Pakistan. *Eastern Mediterranean health journal*, 2003, 9(4):732–40.

80 Kazemi B, et al. Immunization of Balb/C mice by protein fragments of lizard *Leishmania* promastigote. *Pakistan journal of biological sciences*, 2004, 7(10): 1699–709.

81 Kazemi B, et al. Fractionation of lizard *Leishmania* promastigote protein. *Pakistan journal of biological sciences*, 2004, 7(10):1703–5.

82 Naeieni KH, et al. Seroprevalence, incidence and risk factors of Crimean-Congo hemorrhagic fever in Sistan-va-Baluchistan province, Iran. *Iranian journal of public health*, 2004, 33(4):1–7.

83 Abdo-Rabbo A, Bassili A, Atta H. The quality of antimalarials available in Yemen. Malaria journal, 2005, 4(28), doi: 10.1186/1475–2875–4–28.

84 El Sherbini A, et al. Risk factors and diagnostic criteria of brucellosis in an endemic area in Egypt. *Infectious diseases in clinical practice*, 2005, 13(6):295–9.

85 Firooz A et al. Imiquimod in combination with meglumine antimoniate for acute cutaneous leishmaniasis: A randomized assessor-blind controlled trial. *Archives of dermatology*, 2006, 142:1575-9.

86 Kabbash I et al. Pattern of condom use among males in lower Egypt. *Eastern Mediterranean health journal*, 2007, 6:1405–1416.

87 Kabbash I et al. Evaluation of risk perception and precautions taken by health care workers for HIV infection in hemodialysis units. *Eastern Mediterranean health journal*, 2007,13:392–407.

88 Ishag Adam et al. ABO blood group system and placental malaria in an area of unstable malaria transmission in eastern Sudan. *Malaria journal*, 2007, 6:110 doi:10.1186/1475-2875-6-110

89 Kattar M et al. Development and evaluation of real-time polymerase chain reaction assays on whole blood and paraffin-embedded tissues for rapid diagnosis of human brucellosis. *Diagnostic microbiology and infectious disease*, 2007, 59:23–32.

90 Sadeghian G, Nilfroushzadeh MA, Iraji F. Efficacy of local heat therapy by radiofrequency in the treatment of cutaneous leishmaniasis, compared with intralesional injection of meglumine antimoniate. *Clinical and experimental dermatology*, 2007, 32, 371–374.

91 Masjedi MR, Fadaizadeh L, Taghizadeh Asl R. Notification of patients with tuberculosis detected in the private sector, Tehran, Iran. *International journal of tuberculosis and lung disease*, 2007, 11(8):882–886.

92 El Sherbini A et al. Seroprevalences and local variation of human and livestock brucellosis in two villages in Gharbia Governorate, Egypt. *Transactions of the Royal Society of Tropical Medicine and Hygiene*, 2007, 101: 923–928.

93 Rumman KA et al. Prevalence of tuberculosis suspects and their healthcare-seeking behavior in urban and rural Jordan. *The American journal of tropical medicine and hygiene*, 2008, 79:545–551.

94 Bassili A et al. Diagnostic and treatment delay in tuberculosis in 7 countries of the Eastern Mediterranean Region. *Infectious diseases in clinical practice*, 2008, 16:23–35.

95 Mustafa HS et al. Malaria preventive measures, health care seeking behaviour and malaria burden in different epidemiological settings in Sudan. *Tropical medicine and international health*, 2009, 14:1–8.

96 Al-Absi A et al. The decline of tuberculosis in Yemen: evaluation based on two nationwide tuberculin surveys. *International journal of tuberculosis and lung disease*, 2009, 13:1100–1105.

97 Himeidan YE et al. Short report: Permethrin and DDT resistance in the malaria vector *Anopheles arabiensis* from eastern Sudan. *The American journal of tropical medicine and hygiene*, 2007, 77:1066–1068.

Other publications

1 *Diagnostic and treatment delay in tuberculosis: An in-depth analysis of the health seeking behaviour of patients, and health system response in seven countries of the Eastern Mediterranean Region.* Cairo, WHO Regional Office for the Eastern Mediterranean, 2006 (WHO-EM/TDR/009/E).

2 Rakhshani F. *Manual of active teaching skills in malaria education (for health primary care workers).* Zahedan, Zahedan University of Medical Sciences, 2004.

3 ElTigani H. *Training manual for teachers for the detection of malaria among school children.* Khartoum, University of Khartoum, 2004 (Arabic).